Traumatic Injuries of the Genitourinary System

International Perspectives In Urology

Volume 1

Traumatic Injuries of the Genitourinary System

W. Scott McDougal, M.D.

Associate Professor of Surgery (Urology)
Dartmouth Medical School
Hanover, New Hampshire

Lester Persky, M.D.

Professor of Urology
Case Western Reserve Medical School
Cleveland, Ohio

Medical Illustrations by
Barbara N. Rankin, A.M.I.

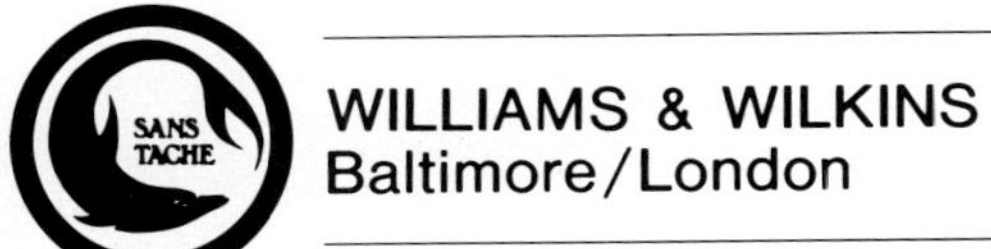

WILLIAMS & WILKINS
Baltimore/London

Copyright ©, 1981
Williams & Wilkins
428 E. Preston Street
Baltimore, MD 21202, U.S.A.

Made in the United States of America

Library of Congress Cataloging in Publication Data

McDougal, William Scott, 1942–
    Traumatic injuries of the genitourinary system.

    Includes index.
    1. Genito-urinary organs—Wounds and injuries. 2. Traumatology. I. Persky, Lester, joint author. II. Title. [DNLM: 1. Urogenital system—Injuries. WJ100 M137t]
RD571.M33   617'.46   80-14976
ISBN 0-683-05768-5

Composed and printed at the
Waverly Press, Inc.
Mt. Royal and Guilford Aves.
Baltimore, MD 21202, U.S.A.

Series Editor's Foreword

The pageant of civilization and the improvement of mankind rests with the intermingling of people through migration and the exchange of ideas. Historically, as a lessor culture establishes contact with a higher culture, it learns from its new neighbors; they furnish it with models, both artistic and practical; they serve as its teachers and by imitation it grows. Mankind is not content with imitation but has moved to emulate its teachers and creates new forms for itself.

International Perspectives in Urology is designed to promote an international exchange of ideas. International authorities in urology will contribute to this series in the hopes that world-wide exchange of ideas will enhance the intellectual growth and development of urology. It is further hoped that the free exchange of urologic ideas will improve the quality of urologic care around the globe.

International Perspectives in urology breaks new ground with the publication of this monograph series. I hope that the series will satisfy the needs of urologists around the world and that the benefits of the international exchange of urologic ideas is realized.

JOHN A. LIBERTINO, M.D.
Series Editor

Preface

Traumatic injuries are rarely isolated to one organ system and therefore, when the genitourinary tract is involved, associated injuries are to be anticipated. The nature of the associated trauma often modifies the type of therapy employed for the urologic injury. Moreover, trauma may cause alterations in the function of the heart, lung, kidney and body metabolism even though these systems have not been directly injured. For these reasons, the Urologic Trauma Surgeon must not only be prepared to diagnose and treat the specific injury, but he must also be able to provide the support necessary so that the vital functions are optimally preserved. The first two chapters deal with general supportive aspects of the care of the trauma patient and the remaining five chapters with the etiology, classification, diagnosis, treatment and complications of specific genitourinary tract injuries. Diagnostic roentgenographs and surgical procedures are illustrated, and it is our hope that the illustrations and text will provide the proper foundation for the complete care of the trauma patient whose injury involves the urologic system.

W. Scott McDougal, M.D.
Lester Persky, M.D.

Contents

CONTENTS

1

Care of the Trauma Patient

INITIAL CARE

The principles of initial management for the urologic trauma patient are identical to those for any injured individual. There is a tendency, however, for the specialist to focus on his particular area of expertise and thereby inadvertently overlook aspects of immediate care which are essential to the patient's survival. Therefore, the urologist must determine that the following aspects of care have been instituted before proceeding to the specific urologic evaluation.

The patient's airway must be clear and respiratory exchange unimpeded. (The management of patients with respiratory insufficiency is described subsequently.) Hemorrhage must be controlled and a large bore intravenous (IV) catheter should be positioned in such a way as to preclude the possibility of an injured vessel lying between the IV entrance site and the heart. For example, it is inappropriate to place a single IV in the femoral vein in a patient who has sustained abdominal trauma. Should the vena cava be injured, the infusate will not reach the heart where it is needed but rather enter the abdomen. Multiple IV's, one of which is centrally placed, are indicated when major vascular injuries have been sustained or when blood loss is considerable. Blood pressure must be maintained, initially with infusions of crystalloid, colloid, or stroma-free hemoglobin and ultimately with type-specific blood, should prior blood loss warrant. A baseline set of laboratory data should be obtained, including a complete blood count, serum electrolytes, glucose, blood urea nitrogen, creatinine, and amylase. Arterial blood gases are obtained when indicated. The patient should also be typed and cross-matched for blood.

The nature of the patient's immunization status for tetanus must be determined. Adult patients are immunologically competent when they have received at least three injections of toxoid, the last within 10 years of the current injury. Children under 7 years of age require four injections

1

of toxoid followed by a fifth at age 4 to 6 years. They are immunologically protected thereafter and require a booster injection at 10 year intervals. Patients who have been fully immunized and who have received a booster within the last 10 years do not require a toxoid injection, provided the wound is not at high risk for tetanus. In those patients whose wounds are prone to *Clostridium tetani* infestation, 0.5 cc of tetanus toxoid is given if their last booster was obtained more than 5 years previously. If the patient has received two or more injections of toxoid, but the last dose was given more than 10 years ago, 0.5 cc tetanus toxoid is administered. All others who have wounds which could harbor *C. tetani* should be given 0.5 cc tetanus toxoid plus 250 units or more of tetanus immune globulin injected at a site distant from the toxoid injection.[1]

A history and physical examination including a neurologic exam must also be obtained. The gravity of the patient's condition dictates the nature of the history and physical, but if initially brief, it must be thorough with respect to the nature and extent of injury as well as with respect to the vital functions provided by the respiratory, neurologic, and cardiovascular systems. As early as is consistent with good care, a complete history and physical must be obtained—a point often overlooked in the care of trauma patients. Finally, fractures should be splinted, and when indicated, a nasogastric tube inserted. It is important to note that the placement of a Foley catheter is not part of the initial management and is performed only after the lower genitourinary tract has been carefully examined (vide infra).

THE UROLOGIC EXAMINATION

Evaluation of the traumatized patient requires a systematic approach. A thorough history is obtained which must include questions directed at determining the presence of bleeding tendencies, prior hematuria, congenital or acquired genitourinary disease, micturition difficulties, urinary tract infections, prior genitourinary trauma, and operative procedures. The physical examination includes observation of the abdomen and flank for symmetry, palpation of the flanks and suprapubic areas for masses, rib fractures, or tenderness, palpation of the pelvic bony structure for fractures, observation of the external genitalia, perineum, and urethral meatus for blood or echymoses, palpation of the penile shaft and testes for tenderness, and rectal examination of the prostate for tenderness and position. Radiographic examination follows the history and physical examination.

The sequence in which diagnostic roentgenographs of the genitourinary system should be obtained proceeds from the urethra to kidney, eliminating those studies which are unnecessary as determined by the history and physical examination. A urethrogram is performed, preferably under fluoroscopic control, by placing a 10 to 14 French Foley catheter in the fossa navicularis and inflating the balloon until a snug fit is obtained. Ten cc of 10 to 20% water soluble radiocontrast is injected. If flouroscopy is not available, the film should be exposed during the injection, for if

TRAUMATIC INJURIES OF THE GENITOURINARY SYSTEM

postinjection films are obtained, coaptation of the urethral walls may prevent visualization of the entire structure. If the urethra is uninjured, a Foley catheter is introduced into the bladder through which 300 to 400 cc of contrast is allowed to flow by gravity. Following the radiograph of the full bladder, the contrast is completely drained from the bladder and another roentgenogram obtained. Some advocate washing the bladder with saline to assure complete removal of all intravesical radiocontrast. The postdrainage film will reduce the chance of missing a small posterior extravasation which might be hidden by the dye-distended bladder. Finally, an IV pyelogram is obtained. Angiography, ultrasonography, and computerized axial tomography follow when indicated.

When several disciplines are involved in the care of the multiply injured patient, the efforts of all must be coordinated into a sequence which is most advantageous for the individual patient. The order in which injuries are repaired is dependent upon priorities of care which are determined by the life-threatening nature of the injury as well as its potential for prolonged morbidity. Moreover, the Urologic Trauma Surgeon must be prepared to adapt his therapy according to the overall needs of the patient. For example, a multiply injured patient with a posterior urethral disruption who is unstable due to other traumatic injuries should not be subjected to a primary repair even though the surgeon may feel this to be optimal therapy for that particular genitourinary injury. Under these circumstances, a suprapubic cystostomy is preferred since it results in little blood loss and requires little operative time, thereby allowing the major thrust of therapy to be directed at the life-threatening injury.

The general care of trauma patients requires that the Urologic Surgeon be knowledgeable about respiratory, fluid and electrolyte, cardiovascular, renal, and blood transfusion complications. Therefore, a brief consideration of the most commonly encountered difficulties follows.

RESPIRATORY DYSFUNCTION

Respiratory Insufficiency

Inadequate ventilation in the post-traumatic and postoperative periods results in hypercapnia or hypoxemia, or both. The primary goal of therapy is to provide the patient with the capability of maintaining an arterial oxygen partial pressure of at least 60 mm Hg on an inspired oxygen content as close to room air as possible. In order to achieve this goal, oxygen delivered by nasal prongs, a face mask, or an endotracheal tube with respirator support may be required. There are, however, constraints to the amount of oxygen which can be delivered. Limitation of the amount may be a consequence of the device used for delivery; however, more commonly, the amount which can be safely delivered is limited by the fact that inhalation of high oxygen concentrations results in pulmonary toxicity. The hazards of high concentrations include suppression of the respiratory drive in patients with chronic lung disease, retrolental fibroplasia—primarily a disease of the newborn, but it has been described in adults—segmental atelectasis due to the greater solubility of oxygen compared to nitrogen, impairment of respiratory ciliary function, decrease in pulmonary surfactant, and direct injury to capillary endothelial cells.

The arterial carbon dioxide partial pressure which is normally 40 mm Hg is a primary indicator of the adequacy of ventilation. Common causes of hypercapnia include obstructive lung disease, adult respiratory distress syndrome, metabolic alkalosis, and respiratory depression due to sedation or central nervous system trauma. Hypocapnia may be a result of hypoxia, anxiety, pulmonary embolism, sepsis, and pulmonary insufficiency. Although an indicator of ventilatory adequacy, alteration of pCO_2 by itself is rarely an indication for respiratory support. Of more importance is the pO_2 which should be maintained above 60 mm Hg. A pO_2 less than 60 mm Hg requires a change in respiratory management. (The normal pO_2 for a particular patient breathing room air prior to injury may be estimated by subtracting one-half the individual's age from 100.)

If impending airway obstruction is not a problem, initial support of the pO_2 may be obtained by the use of nasal prongs or face masks. Humidified oxygen should be used when possible in order to prevent drying of the nasotracheal mucosa. Oxygen delivered by nasal prongs generally cannot provide an inspired concentration much above 50%. Even though humidified, high flows have a drying effect on the mucosa. Venturi masks provide constant flows of oxygen ranging between 24 and 40%, depending upon the mask. Partial rebreathing masks can deliver in excess of 80% oxygen; however, humidity cannot be added to the system.

On occasion, post-traumatic patients require endotracheal intubation—preferably by the nasotracheal route with a prestretched low pressure cuff—and respiratory support. The indications for intubation include: 1) the facilitation of pulmonary toilet, 2) the prevention of upper airway occlusion, 3) a protection against aspiration, and 4) the need for mechanical ventilation (Table 1.1). The requirement for mechanical ventilation is assessed by 1) vital capacity, 2) inspiratory force, 3) respiratory rate, 4) arterial oxygen content, and 5) work of breathing. Vital capacity or the volume of a maximal inspiration following a maximal expiration is normally 60 to 70 ml/kg body weight. If it is less than 15 ml/kg, ventilatory support is indicated. The inspiratory force or the amount of pressure one is able to generate against a closed airway is normally -75 to -100 cm H_2O. Patients who can achieve no more than -25 cm H_2O require mechanical support. The normal respiratory rate is 12 to 20/min.

Table 1.1

Indications for endotracheal intubation

Facilitation of pulmonary toilet
Prevention of upper airway occlusion
Protection against aspiration
Need for mechanical ventilation as determined by
1. A vital capacity less than 15 ml/kg body wt
2. An inspiratory force less than -25 cm H_2O
3. A respiratory rate in excess of 35/min.
4. A pO_2 less than 60 mm Hg despite high ambient O_2 concentrations
5. An excessive and prolonged increase in the work of breathing

TRAUMATIC INJURIES OF THE GENITOURINARY SYSTEM

A rate which exceeds 35 suggests the need for ventilatory assistance. The arterial oxygen partial pressure or pO_2 should exceed 60 mm Hg. If this cannot be accomplished by raising the oxygen content of inspired air through the use of face masks and nasal prongs, intubation should be performed. Severe intercostal retractions and a tracheal tug indicate an increased work of breathing and are forerunners of respiratory insufficiency.

Initially, the respirator is adjusted to deliver 12 to 15 ml/kg body weight at a frequency of 8 to 14 times per minute for the adult and 15 to 30 times per minute for the child. The inspired oxygen content or FiO_2 should be the lowest needed to maintain the pO_2 above 60 mm Hg (an FiO_2 of 40% is a good level to begin with, adjusting it upward or downward as required). Not only must blood gases be monitored, adjusting the respirator accordingly, but the circulatory status must be carefully followed, for on occasion institution of mechanical ventilation will cause a fall in the cardiac output with a resultant lowering of blood pressure. When the pO_2 cannot be maintained by an acceptable FiO_2 (less than 60%), the addition of positive end expiratory pressure (PEEP) may be helpful. This technique maintains a specified pressure at the end of each respiration rather than allowing end expiratory pressure to fall to zero. It is particularly useful in the adult respiratory distress syndrome (vide infra). Initially, 5 cm H_2O pressure is employed. If the desired response is not achieved, it is increased in increments of 5 cm H_2O, carefully monitoring the blood pressure for signs of a significant reduction in cardiac output. Usually, no more than 15 cm H_2O is required; however, on rare occasions as much as 25 cm H_2O may be needed. With the use of PEEP, pO_2 can be maintained at acceptable levels using reduced FiO_2's. Other advantages include a decrease in pulmonary shunting and an increase in functional residual capacity (FRC). A proposed advantage is that it drives pulmonary edema fluid from the alveoli and interstitium into the pulmonary capillaries. Its major disadvantages are a reduction in cardiac output and a diminished urine output. The latter effect is perhaps a result of an increased release of antidiuretic hormone.

One method of anticipating future respiratory difficulties as well as determining how the patient is progressing on the respirator is by sequentially determining the arterial oxygen gradient $(A\text{-}aDO_2)$; this gradient is a sensitive indicator of early respiratory impairment. In order to calculate the $A\text{-}aDO_2$ gradient, the patient is placed on 100% oxygen for 20 to 30 minutes. Arterial blood gases are drawn and the barometric pressure recorded. The calculation is as follows: barometric pressure minus water vapor pressure (47 mm Hg) minus the partial pressure of alveolar CO_2 (because alveolar CO_2 rapidly equilibrates with arterial CO_2, the pCO_2 obtained from the blood gas analysis may be substituted). This quantity minus the pO_2 is equal to the arterial alveolar oxygen gradient. A normal value lies between 25 and 65. A value exceeding 450 suggests failure.

Ventilatory support is continued until the indications for its use no longer apply. If mechanical ventilation was the reason for intubation, the patient may be weaned from the respirator when the chest roentgenogram reveals no deterioration, the spontaneous respiratory rate is less than 30/

minute, PEEP is no longer required, the inspiratory force exceeds -25 cm H_2O, the vital capacity exceeds 15 ml/kg, and the pO_2 can be maintained above 60 mm Hg on a FIO_2 below 50%. The patient is weaned by placing him on a T-piece with humidified oxygen for 10 minutes of each hour. If the T-piece is tolerated, the time on it is gradually increased until the respirator is no longer required. The blood gases and the patient's respiratory effort must be carefully monitored both during weaning and following extubation.

Adult Respiratory Distress Syndrome

Acute post-traumatic pulmonary insufficiency (ARDS) occurs following major trauma, burns, hypoproteinemia or inadequate fluid resuscitation during shock, severe sepsis, pancreatitis or transplantation rejection crisis (antigen-antibody reaction). Following the initiating event, platelet microaggregates form in the pulmonary capillaries and injure the alveolar capillary endothelium. Vasoactive substances are released resulting in increased capillary permeability.[2] Peribronchiolar edema follows which causes an increase in small airway resistance and a reduction in lung compliance making aeration of the lungs difficult. Pulmonary shunting also occurs. The pO_2 falls and the pCO_2 rises, often despite increases in the FIO_2. The oxygen exchange ratio exceeds two (the oxygen exchange ratio is merely the alveolar arterial oxygen gradient divided by the pO_2). Clinically, the patient becomes dyspneic, tachypneic, and hypoxemic. There is a reduced FRC, reduced lung compliance, and often bilateral pulmonary infiltrates are present on the chest film. The syndrome should be suspected in the traumatized patient when the pO_2 falls despite efforts to increase the FIO_2. Treatment involves nasotracheal intubation and mechanical ventilation. PEEP is often necessary. If PEEP results in a reduced cardiac output, inotropic agents may be required in order to return blood pressure to acceptable levels. Isoproterenol, 0.25 to 1.0 μg/ min, glucagon, 3 mg/hr, or digoxin are acceptable. The use of colloid to increase intravascular oncotic pressure and thereby draw fluid from the pulmonary perivascular space into the capillaries is controversial as is the use of steroids. Prophylactic antibiotics administered either by the parenteral route or by inhalation have little to recommend them. Infections are treated when they occur with the antibiotic to which the bacteria are sensitive.

Pulmonary Embolism

Pulmonary emboli may occur silently and be an incidental finding on a chest film, or they may suggest their presence by causing dyspnea, chest pain, hemoptysis, and rarely, when massive, circulatory collapse. On physical examination, the pulmonic portion of the second heart sound may be increased, a parasternal heave may occur, on occasion a friction rub can be heard, and the electrocardiogram often shows right heart strain as evidenced by right axis deviation. Chest x-ray, when positive, reveals a lucent area which lacks vascular markings. Later a wedge-shaped infiltrate develops. Pulmonary scans may be used to support the diagnosis

　　TRAUMATIC INJURIES OF THE GENITOURINARY SYSTEM

but the definitive study is a pulmonary angiogram. Therapy is directed at identifying the source and treating it while simultaneously anticoagulating the patient, initially with a continuous heparin infusion. If the pulmonary embolus is large or saddle in type and is causing circulatory collapse which is unresponsive to supportive measures, a pulmonary embolectomy is indicated.

VOLUME AND ELECTROLYTE BALANCE

Immediate restoration of volume disturbances and electrolyte abnormalities in the traumatized patient is critical if subsequent cardiac, respiratory, neurologic, and renal dysfunction are to be avoided. Hemorrhage must be controlled and blood volume restored. Patients who have lost more than 1500 cc generally require transfusion. A blood loss equal to or exceeding 2% of the body weight results in shock and requires immediate restoration of blood volume. As a temporizing procedure, Ringer's lactate is infused initially at a rate sufficient to return blood pressure to acceptable levels or until such time as blood becomes available. Albumin, stroma-free hemoglobin, starch solutions, and dextran may also be used in limited amounts to maintain intravascular oncotic pressure until blood becomes available. Unfortunately, their excessive use in some shock states where capillary permeability is markedly altered may result in extravascular deposition with worsening of interstitial fluid accumulation. Moreover, infusion of large amounts of dextran alters hemostatic mechanisms and impure stroma-free hemoglobin may lead to acute renal failure.

Large losses are readily appreciated and immediate therapy straightforward; however, as resuscitation continues or when the injury has resulted in cardiac malfunction, sequential assessment of volume status is critical. Blood pressure and urine output are good guides but because of homeostatic mechanisms they provide no more than a gross estimate of volume replacement. The volume status can be more accurately assessed by central venous, pulmonary artery, and left atrial pressure measurements. Central venous pressure (CVP) is a good reflection of volume status provided there is no cardiac dysfunction. It may also be used to guide fluid therapy in those patients with cardiac abnormalities in which both ventricles are equally affected by the disease. Under these circumstances there is a good correlation between CVP and left ventricular filling pressure. Normal values range between 5 and 12 cm H_2O, depending upon the point of reference. We prefer to use the midaxillary line as the reference point since it is easily found and diminishes the chance of error arising from varying reference points when multiple observers perform the measurement. The important point is that CVP should be measured serially from the same reference point, thus allowing a dynamic accurate assessment of the adequacy of resuscitation. A patient with a low CVP should be given fluid until it is within the normal range.

When the CVP does not seem to correlate with blood pressure or in those patients with cardiac disease in which the two ventricles may be disproportionately affected, a more accurate guide is obtained by following pulmonary artery and left atrial pressures. These measurements are made using the Swan-Ganz catheter which is placed percutaneously into a major vein (jugular, subclavian, femoral) and directed into the right heart. The balloon on the tip of the catheter allows it to be floated through the ventricle into the pulmonary artery. Catheter position is determined by the pressure profile (Fig. 1.1) and final placement confirmed by x-ray (Fig. 1.2). The normal pulmonary artery pressure is 9 to 17 mm Hg. If the balloon is inflated in a branch of the pulmonary artery thereby occluding inflow, a pulmonary capillary wedge pressure (PCWP) is obtained which reflects left atrial pressure (normal 5 to 12 mm Hg). Thus, a low pulmonary artery pressure and PCWP indicate the need for volume replacement. If the PCWP is raised to 15 mm Hg without improvement in cardiac output, the need for an inotrope is suggested. With the thermal dilution Swan-Ganz catheters, cardiac output can also be measured. Once the patient's volume status has been restored to normal, maintenance fluid and electrolyte replacement must be calculated.

Maintenance Fluids

The amount of fluid which must be provided to the patient in order to maintain homeostasis is equivalent to the urine output plus insensible loss plus abnormal losses minus the water produced by the metabolism of fat, carbohydrate, and protein (Table 1.2). Each of these entities must be calculated for the individual patient if optimal fluid balance is to be achieved.

The amount of urine necessary to maintain proper balance is dictated by the physiologic limits of the kidney for solute and water excretion. In resting man, the products of normal metabolism produce a solute load which requires a minimum of 400 to 600 cc of urine for excretion. Traumatized and critically ill patients are often hypermetabolic and produce increased solute loads, thereby necessitating slightly greater amounts of urine production. On the other hand, excessive output may lead to a washout of the renal medullary osmotic gradient resulting in

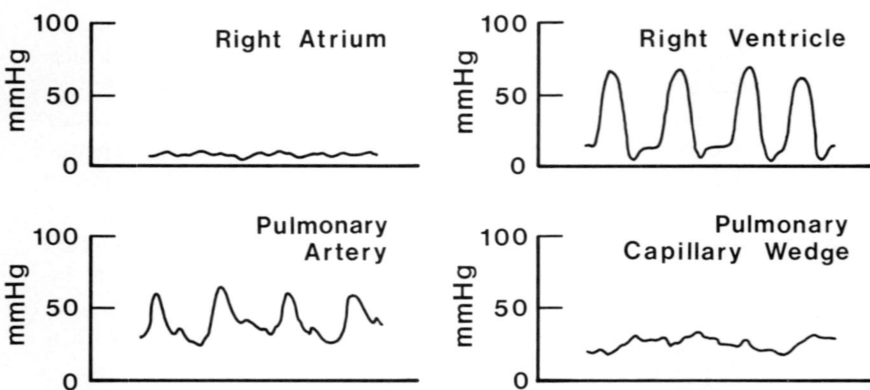

Figure 1.1. Pressure tracings of the right atrium, right ventricle, pulmonary artery, and pulmonary capillary wedge. As the Swan-Ganz catheter is passed through the heart into the pulmonary artery, its position is determined by the pressure tracing and final placement confirmed radiographically.

TRAUMATIC INJURIES OF THE GENITOURINARY SYSTEM

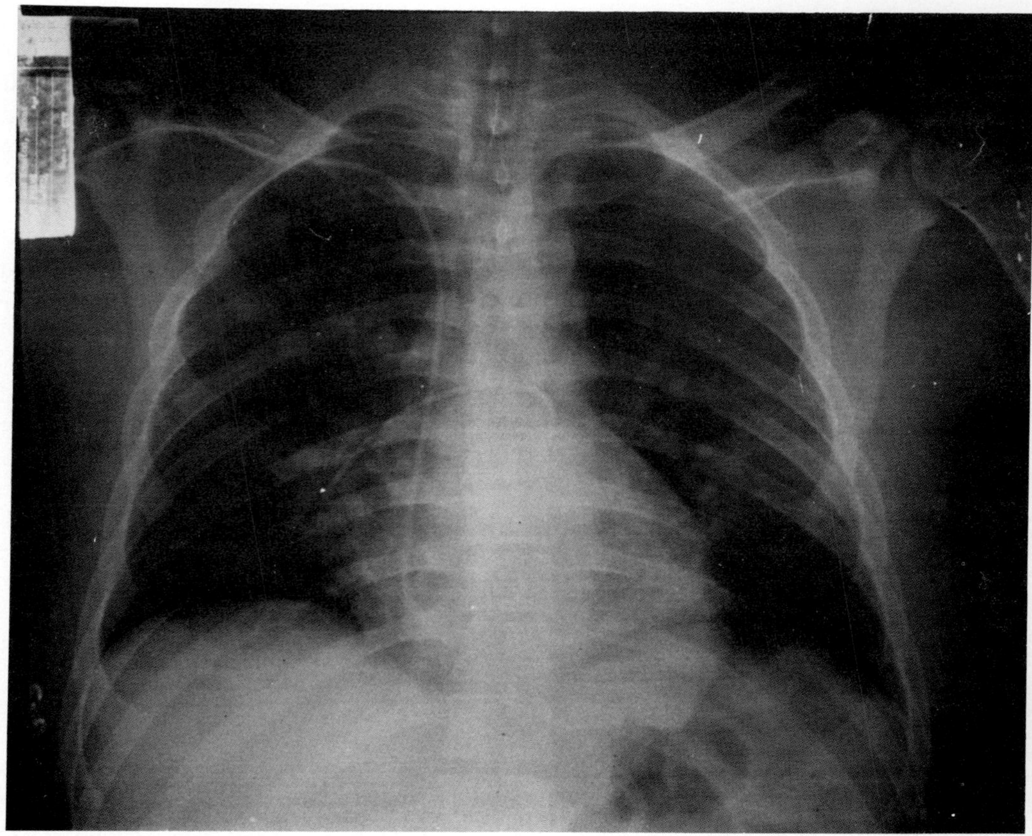

Figure 1.2. Roentgenogram of a Swan-Ganz catheter in position.

Table 1.2
Summary of formulas for fluid administration

Basic fluid requirement	= (U.O. + Insens. + Abn. Loss) − H_2O Met.
Urine Output (U.O.)	= 30-50 cc/hr, adult or 20-40 cc/kg/24 hrs, child
Insensible loss (Insens.)	= 10-15 cc/kg/24 hrs, adult or 45 cc/100 kcal, child
Abnormal loss (Abn. Loss)	= measured external or estimated third space losses
Water of Metabolism (H_2O Met.)	= 10% × (25 × kg body wt), adult or 10% × (kcal metabolized), child

impaired concentrating capabilities of the kidney. The fluid intake required to produce large urine outputs may also result in fluid retention and vascular overload. Therefore, there are limits between which urine output should be maintained. The adult kidney is most efficient in maintaining balance when fluid intake is sufficient to produce a urine output of 800 to 1200 cc/day or 30 to 50 cc/hr. In children, urine output should be maintained between 20 and 40 cc/kg body weight/day. Under

CARE OF THE TRAUMA PATIENT   9

specific circumstances, the urine output may have to be adjusted upward. Patients who have sustained crush or electric injuries in which the nephrotoxic hemochromogen myoglobin is released should have their urine output maintained at diuretic levels (100 cc/hr) until the myoglobin is cleared. If this is not accomplished, the incidence of acute renal failure (vide infra) as a consequence of myoglobin nephrotoxicity will be markedly increased.

Insensible loss refers to the water lost from the respiratory tract and skin. The amount lost is dependent upon the ambient temperature and humidity as well as the patient's surface area and body temperature. The normothermic adult in a comfortable environment loses between 800 and 1000 cc/day (10–15 cc/kg body wt/24 hr). Since children vary considerably in surface area, insensible losses in children are conveniently related to caloric consumption. Thus, a child will lose about 45 cc of water for each 100 kcal metabolized. The amount of calories consumed per day may be calculated by multiplying the body weight by 100 for each of the first 10 kg, by 50 for each of the second 10 kg, and by 20 for each additional kilogram body weight in excess of 20 kg (Table 1.3). Insensible losses increase by about 10% for each degree of temperature elevation above normal.

The water produced by metabolism is calculated from the caloric expenditure of the patient. The amount of water produced in milliliters is numerically equal to 10% of the total amount of kcal consumed. The resting adult metabolizes approximately 25 kcal/kg body weight/24 hr, whereas the child's caloric expenditure is calculated on a graduated basis as described above. Thus, a 70-kg adult will consume 1750 kcal (25 kcal/kg × 70 kg) and thereby produce 175 cc water, whereas a 15 kg child will consume 1250 kcal (10 kg × 100 kcal/kg + 5 kg × 50 kcal/kg) and thereby produce 125 cc water. Since these volumes are small, the water of metabolism is often disregarded in total fluid calculations in patients with functioning kidneys.

Abnormal losses refer to fluids lost either from the body by nasogastric suction, fistula and iliostomy drainage, vomiting and diarrhea, or from the vascular system by third space sequestration (retroperitoneal edema, trauma, ascites, bowel obstruction, *etc.*) The volumes of these losses are measured when external drainage occurs or estimated when sequestration is present and added to the total daily fluid requirements.

The total daily fluid requirement in an adult is calculated by adding the desired urine output, the insensible loss adjusted for temperature

Table 1.3

Caloric requirements (kcal) of patients at rest per kilogram body weight

Children	kcal/kg body wt
First 10 kg (0–10)	100
Second 10 kg (10–20)	50
Each additional kg in excess of 20	20
Adults	25

TRAUMATIC INJURIES OF THE GENITOURINARY SYSTEM

elevations and measured or estimated abnormal losses. By monitoring the patient's urine output and weight, the appropriateness of the calculated fluid requirement may be determined. The patient who is not receiving total caloric replacement should lose approximately one pound per day unless, as in the immediate postoperative or post-traumatic period, obligate third space sequestration of fluid is occurring. If the urine output or weight status is inappropriate, the fluid administered is adjusted upward or downward, accordingly. An example of total fluid replacement calculation follows: 70 kg febrile (38°C) adult with a nasogastric tube draining 300 cc/day would require: 1200 cc urine output (50 cc/hr × 24 hr) plus 1155 insensible loss (15 cc/kg body wt/24 hr × 70 kg + 10% of this quantity for the one degree temperature elevation) plus 300 cc abnormal loss (NG output) for a total of 2655 cc/24 hours.

In children, total fluid replacement may be calculated from the calories metabolized. One cc of fluid is administered for each kcal metabolized. For each kilogram body weight from 1 to 10, 100 kcal are consumed. For each of the second 10 kg body weight (10 to 20 kg), 50 kcal are metabolized and for every kilogram above 20, 20 kcal are consumed (Table 1.3). Thus, a 25-kg child would require 1000 cc for the first 10 kg, 500 cc for the second 10 kg, and 100 cc for the final 5 kg for a total of 1600 cc/day.

Electrolytes

The average adult eating a regular diet receives approximately 70 to 120 mEq sodium, 60 to 80 mEq potassium, 15 to 25 mEq magnesium and 80 to 140 mEq chloride per day. Although the kidney is extremely effective in conserving sodium, since it can reabsorb in excess of 99% of that which is filtered, total renal function is better preserved if enough is administered so that maximum conservation of that which is filtered is unnecessary. Potassium, on the other hand, is not as efficiently conserved and, therefore, must be provided if potassium depletion is to be avoided. In the immediate post-traumatic period, potassium release from injured tissues usually makes exogenous administration unnecessary. Since magnesium is stored, patients who are in good nutritional balance prior to their injury do not require replacement, provided the period of IV therapy will be of rather limited duration. IV electrolyte requirements may be satisfied by providing the adult with 500 cc normal saline or its equivalent (76 mEq sodium and chloride) and 40 mEq potassium chloride/day.

Baseline electrolyte requirements for children are best calculated on the basis of caloric expenditure. Minimal 24-hr requirements are: 3 mEq sodium/100 kcal, 2 mEq chloride/100 kcal and 2 mEq potassium/100 kcal. Thus, the 30-kg child would require 1700 kcal. The sodium requirement is 17 × 3 = 51 mEq, the chloride requirement is 17 × 2 = 34 mEq, and the potassium requirement is 17 × 2 = 34 mEq.

To these basic requirements, abnormal losses must be added. The fluid lost from the body may be analyzed for its electrolyte content, thereby providing accurate replacement (Table 1.4). Fluid which is sequestered in a "third space" generally closely mimics the electrolyte content of plasma and, therefore, can be replaced accordingly.

Table 1.4
Electrolyte content of gastrointestinal drainage (mEq/l)

	Na	K	Cl
Gastric	60	10	90
Jejunum	105	5	100
Ileum	120	10	105
Cecum	80	20	50
Bile	145	5	100
Pancreas	140	4.5	75

Anuria

The fluid and electrolyte requirements for patients who are anephric or anuric are calculated from insensible and abnormal losses. Insensible loss: an adult should receive 10 to 15 cc/kg body weight/24 hr, whereas a child should receive 45 cc fluid/100 kcal expended. The caloric expenditure is estimated on the basis of weight as described above. Part of the fluid is administered as 10% dextrose in water and part as 5% dextrose in 0.2% normal saline. Potassium is generally not administered unless serum studies indicate the need for replacement. Abnormal losses are added to these basic requirements. These calculations are merely estimates of the patient's needs and, therefore, fluid and electrolyte therapy must be continuously adjusted according to serum electrolyte analyses, patient weight and, when appropriate, urine output.

RENAL DYSFUNCTION

Abnormalities in urine flow in the post-traumatic period are often the first indication of impending renal dysfunction. When either an excessively low (less than 600 cc/24 hr) or excessively large (greater than 2000 cc/24 hr) urine output occurs, one should initially suspect a volume disturbance or cardiac malfunction. If, however, the patient is normovolemic and the cardiac output is normal, one must suspect renal dysfunction. Abnormalities which result in inadequate urine volumes (acute renal failure) are considered first followed by those which cause excessive urine outputs (acute polyuric states).

Acute Renal Failure

Acute renal failure in trauma patients has numerous etiologies (Table 1.5). Irrespective of primary cause, it is associated with significant morbidity and mortality and presents as a progressive rise in serum blood urea nitrogen (BUN) and creatinine, often in the face of a falling urine output. Acute renal failure (ARF) is said to be oliguric when the urine output is less than 400 cc/24 hr and nonoliguric when the urine output exceeds this amount. The initial therapy and prognosis of ARF is not only determined by examining the serum chemistries and state of fluid balance but is dependent as well upon the expeditious assignment of the patient to one of the three subdivisions of this disease: pre-, intra- or

Table 1.5
Etiology of acute renal failure in traumatized patients

Prerenal failure
  Excessive nitrogen loads
  Myocardial pump failure
  Intravascular volume depletion

Intrarenal failure
  Occlusion of renal arteries or renal veins
  Disseminated intravascular coagulation
  Parenchymal damage
    Acute pyelonephritis
    Papillary necrosis
      Diabetes mellitus
      Nephroselerosis
      Sickle cell anemia
      Analgesic medications
    Cortical necrosis
  Hepatorenal syndrome
  Vasomotor nephropathy
    Shock
    Sepsis
    Transfusion reactions
    Crush injury
  Tubular toxins
    Drugs
    Myoglobin
    Poisons

Postrenal failure
  Obstruction of the collecting system
    Tumors
    Calculi
    Infections and inflammatory lesions
    Fibrosis
    Blood clots
    Renal papillae

postrenal. It is necessary, therefore, to begin diagnostic procedures which will determine the type of ARF simultaneously with therapy directed at correcting fluid imbalance and electrolyte abnormalities.

Immediate Management of Acute Renal Failure

A careful history and physical examination will often suggest the type of ARF; however, the immediate management of this disease is dictated by the extent of serum chemical aberations and fluid imbalance. Thus, initial steps are directed at defining these abnormalities. An EKG, urine for microscopic and chemical analysis, and serum electrolytes are obtained. If the serum potassium is elevated, the EKG is helpful since it will indicate the rapidity with which the hyperkalemia must be corrected and will serve not only as a baseline against which the success of therapy may be measured but as a direct readout of the approximate potassium concentration during the patient's course. Hyperkalemia results in progressive peaking of the T wave, prolongation of the QRS complex and, at high concentrations, absence of the P wave. When the serum potassium is greater than 7 mEq/l, or when prominent alteration of the cardiogram occurs (particularly when the P wave is absent), immediate reduction in serum potassium is accomplished by infusing hypertonic sodium bicarbonate and/or administration of insulin and glucose in a ratio of 1 unit/ 5 g. The acidosis and hyperkalemia in these patients is partially corrected by bicarbonate which results in a shift of potassium intracellularly with preservation of electroneutrality by concomitant movement of hydrogen ions out of the cell. If some renal function is preserved, potassium secretion is increased in the distal tubule, since bicarbonate reduces the amount of hydrogen ion competing for the common hydrogen-potassium secretory mechanism, thus allowing it increased access to potassium. Glucose and insulin result in movement of potassium into the cell either by binding it during glucose transport or during glycolytic phosphorylation. These mechanisms result in a transitory fall in serum potassium since it moves out of the cell in the former when acidosis recurs and in the latter when substrate has been metabolized. It is important, therefore, to permanently lower the serum potassium by simultaneously employing an ion exchange resin such as Kayexalate (10–20 g po or 50 g by enema, both given with sorbitol) or by peritoneal or hemodialysis. In the usual clinical setting, 2 to 3 hours are required before ion exchange resins show an effect or before dialysis can be instituted. Most commonly, alkalinization, ion exchange resins, and, occasionally, dialysis are all that are required with glucose and insulin being reserved only for those cases in which hyperkalemia is an immediate threat to life.

The state of fluid balance is determined by analysis of intake and output, weight, venous, pulmonary arterial or left atrial pressure, physical examination, and history. Inappropriate intake for the amount of output most often accounts for the imbalance; however, therapeutic maneuvers used to treat electrolyte abnormalities may be contributory as well. Kayexalate, by exchanging sodium for potassium and sodium bicarbonate, can result in excessive sodium loads and fluid retention. When overhydration or hypernatremia become an emergent problem, dialysis is most effective in correcting the disorder. In the usual clinical setting where time is not of the essence, sodium and fluid restriction often suffice. Low venous or pulmonary wedge pressures, clinical signs of dehydration, a history of blood loss and hypotension indicate volume depletion and are treated by the appropriate fluid replacement.

During the acute treatment of hyperkalemia and fluid imbalance, an attempt should be made to define the type of ARF involved. A careful history and physical examination can often be diagnostic. The aseptic and atraumatic passage of a Foley catheter is helpful from both a diagnostic and occasionally a therapeutic point of view. If the patient is capable of spontaneously voiding and the residual is less than 30 cc, the catheter is withdrawn. If the diagnosis remains unclear after these simple maneuvers, a more sophisticated work-up is in order and will include chemical analysis of the urine and serum for sodium, potassium, urea, creatinine and osmolality, and central venous or right atrial pressure determinations.

　　TRAUMATIC INJURIES OF THE GENITOURINARY SYSTEM

IV pyelography is useful in selected cases; however, the degree of renal deterioration is usually of such an extent that visualization does not occur. Indeed, the dye may cause further deterioration of the severely compromised kidney and, therefore, indiscriminate use is to be condemned.[3] Ultrasonography may be helpful in identifying those patients suffering from obstructive uropathy. If the diagnosis is still in doubt, retrograde pyelography is indicated. The characteristics and therapy for each type of ARF are described in detail subsequently.

Prerenal Failure

Prerenal failure occurs when there is an excessive nitrogen load or reduced blood supply to the kidney. The former may result from increased muscle catabolism, blood breakdown within the gastrointestinal tract, or excessive protein alimentation. The latter appears in the presence of volume depletion, congestive heart failure, in valvular heart disease or any disease which causes myocardial pump failure. The serum BUN: creatinine ratio is greater than 10:1 and the CVP and right atrial pressure in volume depletion are low, provided coexisting myocardial disease is not present. The small volume of urine excreted is highly concentrated with a low sodium content (less than 15 mEq/l). The urine urea concentration divided by the plasma urea concentration (U/P urea) is greater than 20:1 and the U/P osmolality greater than 1.5. The renal failure index defined by the ratio of U/P sodium to U/P creatinine ($U/P_{Na}:U/P_{Cr}$) is less than 2.0. The urine sediment may reveal hyaline casts but generally will be free of casts, red and white blood cells (Table 1.6).

The treatment of prerenal oliguria is directed at the primary disease. Efforts are directed at correcting the abnormality which is responsible for the increased nitrogen load, improvement of the failing myocardium, or volume repletion.

Intrarenal Failure

There are many etiologies of acute intrarenal failure; however, tubular injury most often accounts for ARF in traumatized patients. The BUN: creatinine ratio is 10:1 and the CVP is normal or elevated. The urinary sodium concentration exceeds 40 mEq/l with a variable potassium excretion—usually less than 20 mEq/l. The U/P osmolality is less than 1.2 and the U/P urea less than 10. The renal failure index is greater than 2.0. Tubular epithelial cells and tubular epithelial cell casts may be observed in the urine (Table 1.6).

Roentgenograms of the abdomen with laminograms of the kidneys or ultrasonography of the kidneys should be obtained in an effort to determine whether prior renal disease is superimposed on the acute problem. Pre-existing renal disease may be demonstrated by a bilateral or unilateral small kidney, indicative of a vascular or infectious etiology. An enlarged renal outline may imply acute renal vein thrombosis, infiltrative lesions such as myeloma and lymphoma, or obstruction. Renal scans are occasionally helpful in cases of bilateral renal artery thrombosis and may suggest that arteriography should be performed.

Table 1.6
Indices of acute pre-, intra- and postrenal failure

	Normal	Prerenal	Intrarenal	Postrenal
Blood				
CVP	5–8	Low to nl	nl to elevated	nl to elevated
BUN/creatinine	10:1	> 10:1	10:1	10:1 or >
Urine				
Sodium	15–40	< 15 mEq/l	> 40 mEq/l	> 40 mEq/l
Potassium	15–40	Variable	Variable	Variable
Osmolality (Sp. gr. not appropriate)	400–600	> 450 mOsm/l	< 350 mOsm/l	<300 mOsm/l
Volume	800–1200	Low	Variable	Variable Initially low
Urine/blood ratio				
Urea	20:1	> 20:1	< 10:1	< 5:1
Osmolality	1.5–2.0	> 1:5	< 1.2	< 1.0
Renal failure index $U/P_{Na}: U/P_{Cr}$	2.0	< 2.0	> 2.0	> 2.0
Urine-microscopic	0–1 RBC 0–1 WBC Occ. hyaline cast No cellular casts	Occ. hyaline cast	Tubular epithelial casts RBC's, free heme or myoglobin	RBC's, WBC's Malignant cells crystals

Careful fluid balance, the judicious use of ion exchange resins, dialysis, and the administration of a potent diuretic when oliguria occurs are the hallmarks of therapy. The use of furosemide in the treatment of acute oliguric intrarenal failure is controversial. When given, several studies have failed to demonstrate a more rapid recovery, improved GFR, or a reduction in the number of dialyses required except when cardiac decompensation is present. On the other hand, converting an oliguric patient to a nonoliguric status makes subsequent fluid management less cumbersome, especially in the post-traumatic patient. If it is given, a dose of 80 mg is tried—if unsuccessful it is doubled and repeated until finally a bolus of a gram is achieved. One of three responses occur: 1) Oliguria persists. These patients are treated with replacement of net water requirements (insensible loss − water of metabolism + abnormal losses). If a return in urine output does not occur within 21 days, the chance for recovery of renal function is poor. 2) A diuresis ensues, GFR increases, and an immediate reversal in the rise of BUN and creatinine occurs. These patients recover, often obtaining normal renal function. 3) A diuresis occurs, GFR remains low, and BUN and creatinine continue to rise. These patients are treated with replacement of net water loss plus urine output and abnormal losses. Large sodium losses occur during this phase and require replacement. Potassium losses are small, although rarely they may be excessive and require replacement. Appropriate serum potassium concentrations are maintained by restriction of potassium and the use of ion exchange resins and dialysis.

 TRAUMATIC INJURIES OF THE GENITOURINARY SYSTEM

Dialysis plays an important role in the management of these patients. If the BUN is greater than 100 and the creatinine exceeds 12, dialysis is mandatory. Recent evidence suggests that if the BUN is kept below 70, the incidence of sepsis is reduced from 88 to 63%, bleeding from 60 to 36%, and mortality from 80 to 36%[4]. Dialysis may be accomplished either peritoneally (usually not applicable in the trauma patient) or hemically by the use of a Scribner arteriovenous shunt, a MacIntosh double lumen catheter placed into the iliac vein via the saphenous or by placement of Sheldon catheters into the femoral vessels by the Seldinger technique. The latter two methods are useful for a limited number of dialyses; however, should prolonged hemodialysis be required, the Schibner shunt is preferable. The use of hyperalimentation solutions with essential L-amino acids has been shown to improve recovery and reduce the number of dialyses required and is an important therapeutic modality in patients incapable of oral alimentation.[5]

The mortality in this group is high and is reported to be between 25 and 63%. Sixty to 70% of surviving patients exhibiting an acute tubular injury eventually recover sufficient renal function to support life without dialysis.[6]

Postrenal Failure

The etiology of postrenal failure is divided into lower and upper urinary tract obstruction. The lower urinary tract is evaluated in the preliminary treatment as indicated above by the passage of a Foley catheter. The diagnosis for upper urinary tract obstruction is made by ultrasonography[7] and retrograde pyelography. It should be remembered that the indiscriminate instrumentation of the urinary tract must be avoided since sepsis— the most common cause of death in patients with intrarenal ARF—is most often a consequence of genitourinary manipulation. Complete anuria (lower urinary tract obstruction has been ruled out by the introduction of a Foley catheter) demands retrogrades. In addition to obstruction, total anuria may be due to such intrarenal diseases as bilateral renal artery thrombosis, acute glomerulonephritis, cortial necrosis, and the first 12 to 24 hours of acute tubular injury.

These patients are well hydrated, have normal or slightly elevated CVP's, a BUN:creatinine ratio of 10:1 or greater, and a urine microscopic examination which may reveal red cells, white cells, crystals, or malignant cells. Urine sodium concentration is greater than 40 mEq/l and potassium concentration is variable—usually ranging between 20 and 40 mEq/l. The renal concentrating ability is severely impaired and is reflected by a U/P urea of less than 5 and U/P Osm less than 1.0. The renal failure index exceeds 2.0 (Table 1.6).

Therapy is directed at the site of obstruction requiring either that a Foley, a suprapubic cystotomy, a nephrostomy, a cutaneous ureterostomy, or indwelling ureteral catheters may be left temporarily until the metabolic status of the patient is stable enough to permit the appropriate surgical procedure. During the postobstructed period, large quantities of urine are excreted with a low osmolality and a high sodium concentration (50 to 70 mEq/l). These defects are unresponsive to antidiuretic hormone and aldosterone administration.[8] Volume and sodium are replaced as lost. Dextrose 5% in one-half normal saline is usually the appropriate infusion. Potassium losses are therapeutic initially but if prolonged and excessive, replacement of potassium may be necessary later in the course. Sodium and potassium conservation return to normal within 48 to 72 hours; however, the concentrating defect may persist for 7 to 12 days making dehydration a potential danger should fluid be inappropriately restricted. The majority of these patients—if they respond with a diuresis—will go on to recover renal function. If oliguria persists, the obstruction has caused destruction of parenchyma and such patients are managed as described for intrarenal ARF.

Acute Polyuric States

The etiology of excessive urine output may be classified for purposes of diagnosis into one of three categories: postrenal, prerenal, and intrarenal. Postrenal polyuria occurs as a result of chronic partial urinary obstruction or following the release of complete occlusion. The polyuria is characterized by excessive sodium, potassium, and water losses. Treatment involves replacing urinary losses with one-half normal saline until renal function returns to normal (vide supra).

Prerenal polyuria is due to lack of circulating antidiuretic hormone (ADH). In traumatized patients, the most common reasons for lack of ADH include sepsis, pituitary trauma, and volume overload. Prolonged polyuria will result in washout of the medullary osmotic gradient and thereby superimpose an intrarenal component on the original prerenal etiology. Therapy involves correction of the primary disorder, *i.e.* eliminating volume overload or sepsis. In those patients in whom lack of ADH is due to destruction of the pituitary, exogenous ADH administration is the therapy of choice.

Intrarenal polyuria occurs as a result of intrinsic impairment of the concentrating mechanism. This may occur following metabolic derangements such as hypercalcemia, hypokalemia, and renal tubular acidosis, following anatomic abnormalities caused by sickle cell disease, pyelonephritis, polycystic disease, myeloma, amyloidosis, and polyarteritis nodosa, or following renal transplantation, acute, and chronic renal failure. Exogenous ADH administration is not effective in these disorders, and if the primary disease cannot be corrected, therapy is directed at careful fluid replacement, employing CVP, serum osmolality, and body weight measurements as guides to therapy.

CARDIAC DYSFUNCTION

Low Cardiac Output

Inadequate cardiac output may occur as a result of insufficient delivery of volume to the heart or abnormalities of cardiac function. In either case, it is manifested by a fall in systemic blood pressure. Inadequate venous return may result from insufficient circulating volume and is manifested by a low CVP and PCWP or from mechanical interference with venous return as occurs during respirator support, particularly when PEEP is employed. These abnormalities must be eliminated before ascribing a low cardiac output to a malfunctioning myocardium. The latter results in an elevated CVP and/or PCWP. The therapeutic approach involves the use of inotropes. Digitalis, isoproterenal, norepinephrine, glucagon, and dopamine are acceptable. All are arrhythmogenic and, therefore, necessitate careful monitoring of the electrocardiogram during their use. In the post-traumatic patient, dopamine has many advantages. It increases cardiac output, increases renal blood flow, and diminishes peripheral vascular resistance. Five to 10 μg/kg/min is infused initially—the dose subsequently adjusted to provide the desired cardiac output. When dopamine is ineffective, the other inotropes may be tried.

Cardiac Arrhythmias

In the trauma patient extracardiac abnormalities such as acid base disturbances, electrolyte imbalances, and drug overdosage, are commonly the cause of cardiac arrhythmias. Therefore, it is essential to seek out and correct drug and metabolic abnormalities while treating the arrhythmia.

Atrial Premature Contractions (APC's)

APC's are usually benign and require no specific therapy when few in number; however, if they are frequent with coupling intervals which are less than 450 msec they should be treated in order to prevent the subsequent occurence of atrial fibrillation. Either quinidine, 300 mg p.o. q 4 to 6 hr which slows the A-V node, digoxin 0.125 mg IV q 1 hr (until the arrhythmia is terminated or until a dose of 0.5 mg is achieved followed by sequential doses over a 24-hour period to achieve full digitilization) which increases myocardial contractility and slows the AV node, or procainamide, 100 mg IV q 3 to 5 min until the arrhythmia is terminated or a dose of 1 g is achieved, is administered. Procainamide's effects on the heart are identical to those of quinidine.

Paroxysmal Atrial Tachycardia (PAT)

PAT results in a heart rate of 150 to 250/min. This arrhythmia is commonly seen in young patients with no prior history of cardiac disease; or when associated with A-V block, suggests digitalis toxicity. Treatment involves unilateral carotid sinus massage and edrophonium (an anticholinesterase), 10 mg IV. If neither of these techniques are successful, systolic blood pressure may be raised to 160 mm Hg with a vasopressor or, if hemodynamically stable, cardioversion may be tried. If digitalis excess is etiologic, the drug is withdrawn and if the serum potassium is below 4.5, IV potassium may be given to counteract the effects of digitalis.

Atrial Fibrillation (AF)

AF is commonly due to atrial fibrosis secondary to mitral stenosis or hypertensive cardiovascular disease. The importance of this arrhythmia is underscored by the fact that conversion to normal sinus rhythm generally improves cardiac output by 25%. The probability that conversion will be successful is directly correlated to the length of time the patient has had AF. Patients with this arrhythmia should be digitilized if that has not already been done, to control ventricular rate. Quinidine 200 mg p.o. q 2 hr × 5 followed by 200 mg p.o. tid is usually successful. More recalcitrant cases may be electrically cardioverted; however, this modality does not usually lend itself well to application in the traumatized patient.

Atrial Flutter

Atrial flutter is characterized by an atrial rate of 250 to 350 per minute and is a consequence of atrial fibrosis or pulmonary disease. Therapy involves digitalization.

Ventricular Premature Contractions (VPC's)

This arrhythmia may occur in patients without cardiac disease. VPC's need not be treated if they are infrequent, the patient is asymptomatic, and if there is no prior history of cardiac disease. In patients with heart disease in whom there are more than 6 VPC's per minute or in patients in whom they occur in runs, the arrhythmia should be treated. Quinidine, 200 to 300 mg p.o. q 4 to 6 hr, procainamide, 100 mg IV q 3 to 5 min not to exceed a total dose of 1 g, or lidocaine, 100 to 200 mg IV q 3 to 5 min not to exceed a total dose of 1 g are administered until the arrhythmia is terminated or until the maximal dose is given, whichever occurs first. Diphenylhydantoin or propranolol may also be used.

Ventricular Tachycardia

The rapid heart rate of 100 to 250 beats per minute results in inadequate ventricular filling and reduced cardiac output. This arrhythmia requires immediate treatment with an IV bolus of 100 − 200 mg lidocaine or 100 mg procainamide. The IV bolus may be repeated as necessary until a total dose of 1 gm is administered. A lidocaine drip may be necessary to maintain normal sinus rhythm. Quinidine, propranolol, and cardioversion are also effective.

Ventricular Fibrillation

This arrhythmia is a medical emergency and the patient will die for lack of an adequate cardiac output if normal activity is not restored immediately. Lidocaine, 100 to 200 mg IV may be tried but often cardioversion, 100 to 200 watt seconds, is necessary.

TRANSFUSION REACTIONS

Massive Transfusion

Patients who receive more than 5 units of blood over a short interval may develop acidosis, cardiac arrhythmias, hypothermia, microembolic

TRAUMATIC INJURIES OF THE GENITOURINARY SYSTEM

capillary occlusion, or bleeding diatheses. Acidosis can become particularly severe when more than 20 units of bank blood are infused. Each unit of stored bank blood has a base deficit of 8 mEq and, therefore, 1 ampule of sodium bicarconate (50 mEq) should be given for every 5 units of blood administered. Ventricular fibrillation may occur as a consequence of acidosis but more commonly is the result of hypothermia due to the infusion of cold blood. Therefore, patients receiving large amounts of blood should have it passed through a warmer in order to prevent this complication. Microemboli are prevented by passing the blood through a millipore filter. Filters of less than 40 μm in size may remove platelets and, therefore, the platelet count must be carefully monitored. Bleeding diatheses in the massively transfused may be due to factor deficiencies, disseminated intravascular coagulopathy (DIC) or thrombocytopenia. Since factors V and VIII are poorly preserved in stored bank blood, these factors may be deficient. However, recent evidence suggests that the lack of hemostasis following transfusions which exceed one and one-half of the blood volume is generally due to a platelet deficiency rather than a factor deficiency.[9] The partial thromboplastin time (PTT) and prothrombin time (PT) are obtained to screen for factor deficiencies. The platelet count is diagnostic for platelet deficiency. Measurement of fibrinogen and fibrin split product levels are helpful in determining if the low platelet count is a consequence of DIC. Factor deficiencies are treated with cryoprecipitate or the specific factor and platelet deficiencies are remedied with platelet transfusions. The treatment of DIC is controversial. The simultaneous infusion of heparin and epsilon amino caproic acid has been advocated; however, several series report superior results when therapy is directed at the underlying cause and heparin is deleted from the therapeutic regimen.

Transfusion Reactions

About 60% of all patients receiving blood will have a transfusion reaction. Many reactions, such as isosensitization of the recipient to blood antigen, are not readily recognizable. Those which are clinically significant include allergic reactions, febrile reactions, bacterial contamination resulting in sepsis, and hemolytic transfusion reactions. Allergic responses are manifested by puritis, urticaria, chills, and occasionally bronchospasm. Treatment involves stopping the infusion and administration of an antihistamine (Benadryl, 50 mg). Patients who develop bronchospasm should be given 0.3 to 0.6 mg epinephrine and/or 100 mg of hydrocortisone. Febrile reactions are treated by stopping the infusion and administering an antipyretic. Bacterial contamination may result in sepsis. Therapy involves broad spectrum antibiotics, respiratory and cardiovascular support. Hemolytic transfusion reactions are manifested by chills, fever, chest pain, lack of hemostasis, and dyspnea. A spun blood sample will reveal hemolysis. If the hemolytic transfusion reaction occurs during an operative procedure, a change in the appearance of the blood in the wound to a darker color and an increase in bleeding from the wound edges suggest the complication. Treatment involves discontinuing the transfusion and volume expansion. A diuresis is promoted until the hemoglobin is cleared from the serum.

REFERENCES

1. Committee on Trauma of the American College of Surgeons. A guide to prophylaxis against tetanus in wound management, 1979 revision. *Bull. Am. Coll. Surg.,* July, 1979.
2. Blaisdell, F. W. Pathophysiology of the respiratory distress syndrome. *Arch. Surg. 108:* 44, 1974.
3. Carvallo, A., Ralsowski, T. A., Argy, W. V., Jr., et al. Acute renal failure following drip infusion pyelography. *Am. J. Med. 65:*38, 1978.
4. Conger, J. D. A controlled evaluation of prophylactic dialysis in post traumatic acute renal failure. *J. Trauma 15:*1056, 1975.
5. Abel, R. M., Beek, C. H., Jr., Abbott, W. M., et al. Improved survival from acute renal failure after treatment with intravenous essential L-amino acids and glucose. *N. Engl. J. Med. 228:*695, 1973.
6. Flamenbaum, W. Pathophysiology of acute renal failure. *Arch. Intern. Med 131:*911, 1973.
7. Dhar, S. K., Chandraselshar, H., and Smith, E. C. Renosonographic diagnosis of renal failure. *Clin. Nephrol. 7:*15, 1977.
8. McDougal, W. S., and Wright, F. S. Defect in proximal and distal sodium transport in post-obstructive diuresis. *Kidney Int* et al. *2:*304, 1972.
9. Counts, R. B., Haisch, C., Simon, T. L., et al. Hemostasis in massively transfused trauma patients. *Ann. Surg. 190:*91, 1979.

2

Metabolism and Nutrition in the Traumatized Patient

METABOLISM

Basal Metabolic Rate

Uninjured man at rest expends a definable amount of energy to perform physiologic work, *i.e.* the work required to maintain cardiac output, endocrine function, body temperature, liver function, respiration, renal function, *etc.* The amount of energy required to maintain these functions at rest is called basal metabolic rate and is expressed in calories per hour per square meter of body surface. Since basal metabolism is the energy expended by the cells which constitute the active mass of the body, fat, extracellular fluid, and bone make no direct contribution to the metabolic rate.

The energy used in physiologic work is derived from chemical energy which, in the course of the performance of the work, is converted to heat and lost from the body. Therefore, the basal metabolic rate or energy expenditure may be determined by direct calorimetry in which the heat lost from the body is directly measured. Direct calorimetry is difficult to perform and often impractical in the critically ill patient. Therefore, indirect methods of estimating the basal metabolic rate are more commonly employed. The heat loss may be indirectly estimated from 1) oxygen consumption, carbon dioxide production, and nitrogen excretion; 2) measurement of energy intake and losses coupled with the measurement of changes in body composition; or 3) measurement of insensible water loss, assuming that this represents 25% of the total heat lost.

The basal metabolic energy requirement is dependent upon age, sex, and lean body mass. A 1-month-old infant requires about 40 kcal/day. The requirement increases with age and body mass so that boys between

15 and 18 years consume 1700 kcal/day and girls between 12 and 18 years require 1400 kcal/day. The energy requirement remains relatively stable during the active years of adult life; however, with progressive aging it decreases to 1300 kcal/day for men and 1100 kcal/day for women.[1] The difference in metabolic rate between men and women probably relates to the fact that women have a larger proportion of fat per unit body weight. Indeed, if basal metabolic rate is expressed per unit fat free body weight, it is remarkably similar for both males and females over an age span of 20 to 60 years (1.3 kcal/hr/kg).

Hypermetabolism

The response to injury is characterized by an increase in the basal metabolic rate even though the patient remains at rest. The intensity of this hypermetabolic response is dependent upon the severity of the injury, the nutritional status of the patient, and the presence or absence of infection. Patients in good nutritional balance undergoing an elective operation will change their metabolic rate by no more than 10% in the postoperative period provided there are no complications. In contrast, patients with multiple fractures will increase their resting energy expenditure by 10 to 25%, those with major infections by 20 to 50%, and those with major thermal burns by 50 to 125% (Fig. 2.1). In the early post-traumatic period, satisfaction of these energy demands results in degradation of body protein (manifested by a negative nitrogen balance), depletion of energy reserves, and loss of body weight. The initial catabolic response, in which body protein, fat, and carbohydrate are depleted, is

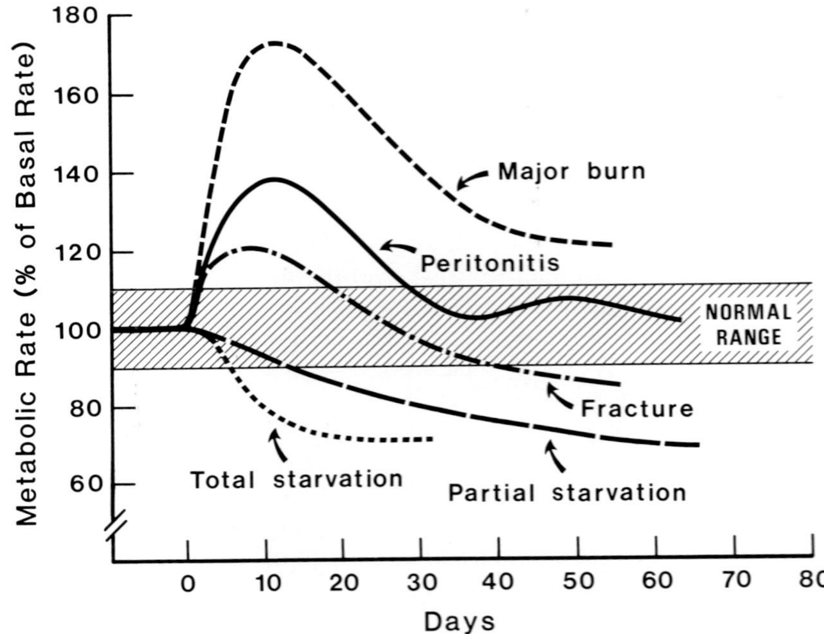

Figure 2.1. Metabolic rate as a function of days postinjury for various types of trauma.

   TRAUMATIC INJURIES OF THE GENITOURINARY SYSTEM

gradually reduced and finally reversed later in the recovery period. An anabolic phase ensues, provided adequate nutritional intake occurs, in which new protein is laid down and during which carbohydrate and fat reserves are repleted. The hypermetabolic response also gradually diminishes as the wounds heal and as infection is eradicated.

In the early postinjury period, energy requirements are satisfied by glucose derived mainly from liver and muscle glycogen and by fatty acids released from adipose tissue. Glycogen reserves are rapidly depleted (usually within 48 hours); however, fat stores which supply the bulk of the energy requirement during this period continue to supply fatty acids for many days. Protein catabolism also occurs, even though it may not serve as a primary energy source. The amino acids released primarily from skeletal muscle are essential for maintenance of cellular metabolism. Moreover, the gluconeogenic amino acids serve as a source for new glucose and provide the basic glucose structure which is necessary for normal metabolism. Rapid depletion of glucose stores coupled with inability of the two carbon fragments of the fatty acids to serve as a source for gluconeogenesis, make protein the only available substrate from which new glucose can be synthesized. Protein catabolism can be reduced but not eliminated by providing the patient with exogenous glucose ("nitrogen sparing effect of glucose").

Catecholamines and Glucocorticoids

Post-traumatic catecholamine levels are elevated (Fig. 2.2) and promote hepatic glycogenolysis, inhibition of insulin release, stimulation of glucagon production and stimulation of fat hydrolysis with the release of free fatty acids. This hormone is produced by the adrenal medulla almost exclusively and has been implicated as the mediator of the hypermetabolic response in injured patients.[2]

The glucocorticoids are also characteristically elevated and remain so throughout the recovery period. The increased production is a direct result of increased ACTH secretion by the anterior pituitary. It is presumed that the pituitary is stimulated to release ACTH by the action of nerves from the periphery responding to the traumatic injury and perhaps by a direct effect of the elevated epinephrine levels. Patients who have sustained severe trauma which requires a prolonged period of convalescence, as in thermal burns, often demonstrate a marked adrenal hyperplasia. Glucocorticoids promote gluconeogenesis and are inhibitory to the action of insulin.

Insulin

In the immediate postinjury period circulating levels of insulin and glucose are elevated. Insulin facilitates glucose transport across cell membranes and inhibits both the release of amino acids from muscle and the release of free fatty acids from adipose tissue. In the post-traumatic period, hyperglycemia is commonly observed and it has been suggested that this is due to the development of insulin resistance by the patient. Indeed, glucose tolerance curves performed during this period simulate

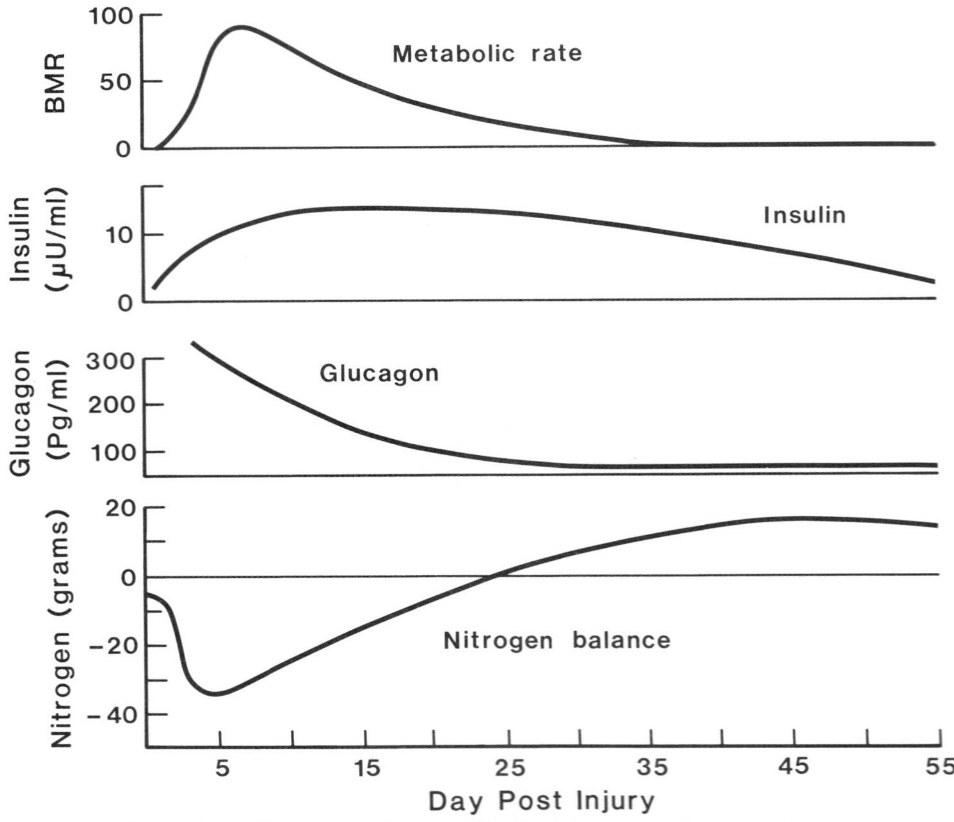

Figure 2.2. Hormonal changes following trauma as a function of days postinjury.

those oberved in diabetes, and have led many to refer to this state as the "diabetes of injury".[3] The mechanism of the hyperglycemia, however, may not be one of insulin resistance. More recent evidence indicates that glucose oxidation is unimpaired and that the hyperglycemia is due to an increase in gluconeogenesis rather than a reduction in peripheral utilization. Moreover, glucose flow studies have clearly demonstrated that the glucose turnover rate is increased above normal.[4, 5]

Glucagon

The increased production of catecholamines postinjury is known to stimulate the alpha cell of the pancreatic islets resulting in increased circulating levels of glucagon, a hormone which promotes glycogenolysis and gluconeogenesis. The relationship between the concentration of insulin and glucagon (the insulin:glucagon molar ratio) determines whether the major influence is toward glucose breakdown or glucose formation. In the early postinjury period, although insulin is elevated, glucagon is disproportionally increased and the ratio of the two favors gluconeogenesis at the expense of protein formation. As healing occurs, the molar ratio reverses, favoring glycolysis and protein formation (Fig. 2.2).

The hypermetabolic response and hormonal balance postinjury direct

TRAUMATIC INJURIES OF THE GENITOURINARY SYSTEM

the metabolism and utilization of carbohydrate, fat, and protein. They set
the stage for a negative nitrogen balance and weight loss, both of which
are related to the extent of injury. The protein which is catabolized to
satisfy energy and substrate requirements is derived mainly from skeletal
muscle. Alanine and glutamine released from the muscle are transported
to the liver where they are converted to glucose (gluconeogenesis). With
protein breakdown, urinary excretion of nitrogen (predominately as urea),
potassium, phosphate, creatinine, magnesium, zinc, and sulfate are markedly increased and reflect catabolism of protoplasmic mass.

NUTRITION

The metabolic response to injury is characterized by hypermetabolism
and hypercatabolism which results in increased tissue breakdown and loss
of essential intracellular constituents. Unlike chronically starved, unstressed individuals, traumatized patients do not adapt to diminished
nutrient intake to conserve protein and energy. Indeed, if exogenous
calories are not provided, seriously injured man catabolizes 200 to 250 g
of body protein daily to satisfy metabolic requirements. Superimposed
infection increases protein loss to 250 to 300 g/day.[6] If this catabolic
response is allowed to persist, decreased immunocompetence, diminished
resistence to infection, impaired wound healing, limitation of vital organ
function, and loss of intestinal enzymes occur.[7-9]

Loss of body protein is the critical factor which determines the point at
which the nutritional depletion compromises the ability of the host to
respond appropriately to the injury. Mortality and morbidity associated
with weight loss and starvation are directly related to loss of essential
protein stores, death occurring with the loss of one-fourth to one-third of
body nitrogen.[10] Therefore, it is essential to limit and ultimately reverse
the loss of body protein in order to reduce the incidence of life threatening
complications and promote early recovery.

In the post-traumatic period, the type, the amount, and the route of
administration are determined by the current nutritional status of the
patient, the degree of hypermetabolism engendered by the trauma, and
the status of the patient's gastrointestinal tract.

Nutritional Status of the Patient

The presence and degree of malnutrition are based on an evaluation of
fat, skeletal muscle, and visceral protein (liver, heart, gut, kidney, *etc.*)
stores. For purposes of estimating the amount of calories required to
restore the patient to a well nourished state, the degree of malnutrition is
graded as mild, moderte, or severe (Table 2.1).

A measure of recent weight loss will indicate the status of the fat and
skeletal muscle mass. If the patient has recently lost less than 10 pounds,
he is said to be mildly malnourished. A 10 to 20 pound weight loss
indicates moderate malnutrition and a weight loss greater than 20 pounds
suggests severe malnutrition. Fat stores can be specifically evaluated by
measuring arm skinfold thickness and comparing the figure to a nomo-

Table 2.1
Classification of malnutrition as mild, moderate, and severe according to weight loss, lymphocyte count, and serum albumin level

Degree of Malnutrition	Recent Weight Loss	Lymphocyte Count	Serum Albumin
	lb	*/mm³*	*g %*
Mild	< 10	1500	3.0 to 3.4
Moderate	10–20	1200–1500	2.5 to 3.0
Severe	> 20	< 1200	< 2.5

gram. Similarly, muscle mass may be individually determined by measuring mid arm circumference and comparing the result to a nomogram. Another measure of muscle protein status may be obtained by determining the 24-hour urine creatinine excretion, dividing the result by the patient's height, and comparing the figure to published tables in which the values for normal men and women are described (Table 2.2). A value less than 75% of predicted normal indicates severe muscle wasting.

The visceral protein status is evaluated by determining the serum albumin level, the lymphocyte count, the serum transferin level, or the patient's ability to recall skin test antigens. A serum albumin level between 3.0 and 3.4 g% indicates mild malnutrition, a level between 2.5 and 3.0 g% moderate malnutrition and a level less than 2.5 g% severe malnutrition. Lymphocyte counts less than 1500/mm³ and serum transferin levels less than 170 indicate malnutrition. Finally, anergy to recall skin test antigens (dermatophyton, *Candida*, varidase, mumps, PPD) indicates malnutrition. In practice, the nutritional status is conveniently determined by measurement of weight loss, lymphocyte count, and albumin level.

Energy and Nutrient Requirements of the Injured Patient

The caloric requirements are ideally determined by indirect calorimetry; however, this is usually not practical in most clinical settings. The caloric requirement may be estimated by adding the basal level of expenditure to that required for hypermetabolism. The basal resting caloric requirement is determined by multiplying the patient's weight in kilograms by 25 kcal. The additional amount due to hypermetabolism ranges between 5 and 60 kcal/kg body weight. An amount is chosen which reflects the severity of injury since the degree of hypermetabolism most closely correlates with the extent of trauma (Fig. 2.1).

Carbohydrate provides about 4 kcal/g and serves as a convenient source of energy. The quantity of carbohydrate administered depends upon the caloric intake desired and the amount of protein administered. Protein provides 4 kcal/g and should be given in amounts of 60 to 100 g or more per day. The calorie to protein nitrogen ratio in a regular diet is about 300 to 1; however, for the critically ill, the amount of protein should be increased to achieve a ratio of 100 to 150 to 1. There is no fat requirement over the short term; however, because of its high caloric density (9 kcal/g), it serves as an excellent energy source. Over the long term, essential fatty acid deficiencies occur if it is not administered. Both

TRAUMATIC INJURIES OF THE GENITOURINARY SYSTEM

water and fat soluble vitamins, trace minerals and electrolytes must also be supplied. The requirements for vitamins and minerals have not been quantitatively determined for the critically ill patient but current information indicates that at least some of them are required in excess of the minimum daily requirements established for healthy man.

To determine the type of nutrient regimen, the caloric requirement is estimated by determining the basal expenditure plus the amount required for the level of hypermetabolism plus an additional amount which will correct the state of malnutrition. Knowing the calorie requirement and the integrity of the gut for alimentation, the proper route or routes may be chosen.

Three routes for nutrient administration are available: 1) enteral, 2)

Table 2.2

Ideal weight and creatinine height index as a function of height for men and women

Height			Medium Frame Ideal Weight		Creatinine/ cm Body Ht/24 hr
ft	*inch*	*cm*	*lb*	*kg*	
			Men		
5	2	157.5	124	56	8.17
5	3	160	127	57.6	8.28
5	4	162.6	130	59.1	8.36
5	5	165.1	133	60.3	8.40
5	6	167.6	137	62	8.51
5	7	170.2	141	63.8	8.62
5	8	172.7	145	65.8	8.76
5	9	175.3	149	67.6	8.86
5	10	177.8	153	69.4	8.98
5	11	180.3	158	71.4	9.11
6	0	182.9	162	73.5	9.24
6	1	185.4	167	75.6	9.38
6	2	188	171	77.6	9.49
6	3	190.5	176	79.6	9.61
6	4	193	181	82.2	9.80
			Women		
4	10	147.3	101.5	46.1	5.63
4	11	149.9	104	47.3	5.68
5	0	152.4	107	48.6	5.74
5	1	154.9	110	50	5.81
5	2	157.5	113	51.4	5.87
5	3	160	116	52.7	5.93
5	4	162.6	119.5	54.3	6.01
5	5	165.1	123	55.9	6.09
5	6	167.6	127.5	58	6.23
5	7	170.2	131.5	59.8	6.32
5	8	172.7	135.5	61.6	6.42
5	9	175.3	139.5	63.4	6.51
5	10	177.8	143.5	65.2	6.60
5	11	180.3	147.5	67	6.69
6	0	182.9	151.5	68.9	6.78

peripheral parenteral, and 3) central parenteral. The most convenient and effective nutritional support is by the enteral route. Often the lack of gastrointestinal motility or the inability to administer large caloric loads by this route will necessitate parenteral administration as supplemental or as the sole source of support. Modest caloric loads may be administered isosmotically by peripheral vein. Large caloric loads given intravenously must be administered centrally since they are hyperosmotic.

The success of the regimen is measured by following the changes in serum albumin, lymphocyte count, serum transferin level, weight and recall skin tests. Although these measurements provide a rough estimate of the efficacy of the regimen, nitrogen balance is the final determinant. An estimate of nitrogen balance may be performed by measuring the urea nitrogen excreted per 24 hours and multiplying the quantity by 1.25 (80% of urinary nitrogen appears as urea) and adding to this value the amount of fecal nitrogen excretion. This quantity is subtracted from the nitrogen taken in. The calculation is made simple when the nutrients are all given by vein since stool measurements become unnecessary.

Enteral Feedings

Because eating patterns have been well established preinjury, most severely traumatized patients allowed ad lib consumption will achieve only 60% of their caloric requirements. Therefore, frequent supplements and continued encouragement by the staff are necessary if optimal caloric consumption is to be achieved. A diet high in calorie and protein content is ideal with supplements administered frequently between meals. There are two types of supplements in general use: those which require digestion and those which require minimal digestion, thereby bypassing the need for most of the pancreatic and biliary secretions ("elemental" diets). Ensure and a calcium casenate formula plus dextrins, medium chain triglyceride oil, egg white powder, other powdered protein sources, whole fresh eggs and flavoring are examples of the former group. The "elemental" group, of which Vivonex is an example, contain carbohydrate in the form of glucose, sucrose, or dextrins, and nitrogen in the form of L-amino acids or acid hydrolysates of casein with amino acids added to provide a balanced pattern. Most "elemental" diets, although low in fat contain essential fatty acids, vitamins, trace minerals, and electrolytes. A high nitrogen elemental diet is commercially available and may be used for patients who are severely depleted. Unfortunately, the elemental diets are not palatable and when used as supplements often require insertion of a small feeding tube for administration. The elemental diet is administered by continuous drip, while the patient eats around the tube.

Tube Feedings

Patients who will not eat or consume insufficient quantities require feeding by tube in order to achieve optimal caloric balance. Since 3000 kcal/24 hr is usually the maximum amount which can be administered when tube feedings are the sole caloric source, oral alimentation in addition is greatly encouraged. The diets administered include high caloric

TRAUMATIC INJURIES OF THE GENITOURINARY SYSTEM

protein supplements such as Ensure, "elemental" products, or blendarized house diets with addition of protein powder, dextrins, fresh eggs, and vitamins. These diets are generally administered with a caloric density of 1 kcal/cc and therefore are hypertonic. Additional water must be administered with tube feedings if dehydration is to be avoided. The feedings should be begun in dilute form and administered every 3 to 4 hours until the proper volume per 24 hours is achieved. The gastric contents should be aspirated before each feeding and replaced. If the gastric return is excessive, the feeding is omitted. The nutrients are administered only when gastric residual remains below 75 cc prior to each feeding. Once volume has been achieved, osmolality (caloric density) may be increased in 30 mOsm increments until 1 kcal/cc is achieved. Higher caloric densities are poorly tolerated. Complications of tube feedings include dehydration with elevated plasma osmolality, gastric distension, diarrhea, cramps, bloating, and aspiration. These complications can be averted by administering the tube feeding only when aspiration prior to each scheduled feeding reveals acceptably low residuals and by carefully monitoring the fluid balance with appropriate addition of water and manipulation of the osmotic content of the feeding as dictated by the state of hydration, plasma osmolality and electrolyte status.

Peripheral or Isosmotic Intravenous Nutrition

Carbohydrate, protein, and fat substrates may be infused individually or in combination in near isosmotic concentrations. Because of their isosmotic character, not only may they be administered by peripheral vein, but the rate of administration may be rapidly changed to satisfy changing fluid requirements or indeed stopped so that medications, colloid, and blood may be administered. These properties make such solutions advantageous during periods of critical care when instability of the patient is common. An understanding of the metabolic effects of each type of caloric source with respect to energy provision, potential for endogenous protein preservation and maintenance of optimal organ function is essential if the proper substrate or combination of substrates is to be administered to acutely ill patients.

The provision of glucose in doses up to 100 g/day decreases the loss of urinary nitrogen. This "protein sparing effect" is directly proportional to the quantity of calories administered. Infusion of larger quantities of glucose results in disproportionately lesser reductions in nitrogen losses. Supplying 700 protein-free calories to fasted normal man results in maximal reduction of protein losses. Increasing the nonprotein caloric intake is without further effect in the sparing of body protein. Indeed, positive nitrogen balance cannot be achieved even with high dose glucose infusions. Starved unstressed man, given approximately 700 g of glucose maintains a negative nitrogen balance of about 1.5 g/m^2/day. However, if the same total caloric load is given but part of the glucose calories are replaced by an equivalent amount of amino acid calories, the negative nitrogen balance is eliminated.[11] Supplying dietary protein with calories further improves nitrogen balance. Thus, on a fixed adequate protein intake energy level is the deciding factor in nitrogen balance and at a fixed adequate caloric intake, nitrogen intake is the determinate of nitrogen balance.[12] Similarly, in critically ill, traumatized patients and in those with superimposed bacteremia, at low dose levels (or those which can be easily achieved employing isosmotic solutions), glucose has the same effect on nitrogen sparing as does an equivalent caloric load of amino acids[6] (Figs. 2.3 and 2.4). Thus, at low dose levels, total caloric load irrespective of whether the calories are derived from protein or carbohydrate determines the degree of nitrogen sparing, whereas when the caloric load is increased, amino acid intake becomes a more dominant determinate of nitrogen balance.

It should be noted, however, that not all are in agreement with the concept that at low dose levels, glucose and amino acids provide the same effect, calorie for calorie, on nitrogen sparing. Blackburn and associates[13] have reported that infusion of intravenous amino acids achieves superior nitrogen sparing only when glucose is omitted from the infusate. However, the data from starved unstressed man and severely stressed thermally injured and septic man demonstrate no difference between glucose and amino acids upon nitrogen sparing when administered at the usual hypocaloric levels normally given injured and postoperative patients. Moreover, exclusion of glucose from the diet is detrimental to normal hepatic and renal function in the severely stressed hypermetabolic patient.[9]

Fat emulsions may also be administered by peripheral vein and have the advantage of providing high caloric loads in relatively small volumes

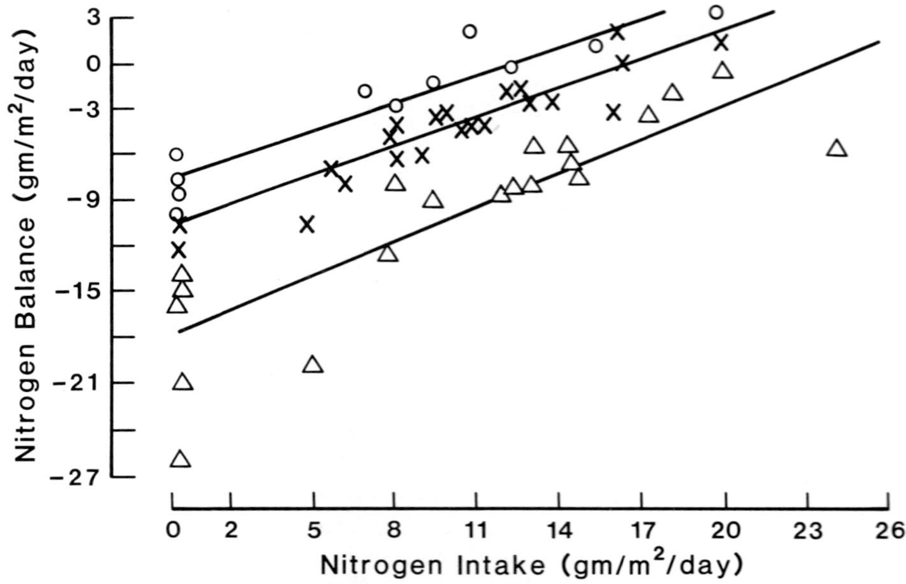

Figure 2.3. Nitrogen balance in nonbacteremic traumatized patients as a function of increasing caloric amounts of amino acids and amino acids plus 60 or 120 g glucose. △, Amino acids without glucose addition; ×, amino acids plus 60 g glucose; ○, amino acids plus 120 g glucose.

 TRAUMATIC INJURIES OF THE GENITOURINARY SYSTEM

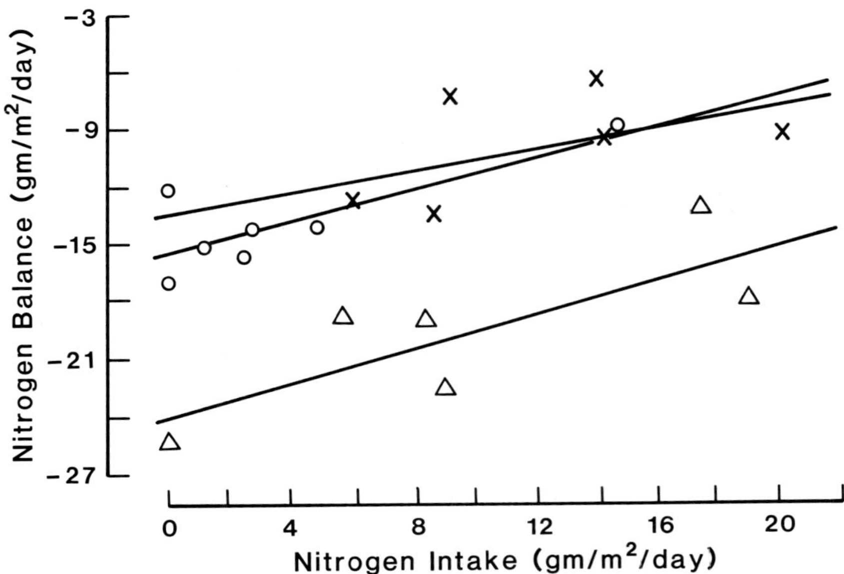

Figure 2.4. Nitrogen balance in bacteremic traumatized patients as a function of increasing caloric amounts of amino acids and amino acids plus 60 or 120 g glucose. △, Amino acids without glucose addition; ×, amino acids plus 60 g glucose; ○, amino acids plus 120 g glucose.

since fat provides 9 kcal/g, whereas glucose and protein provide only 4 kcal/g. The effect of fat emulsions on nitrogen sparing, however, is not equivalent to equal caloric amounts of glucose or amino acids. In normal, unstressed man, equivalent caloric amounts of infused fat emulsion and glucose result in a lesser degree of nitrogen sparing for the former. When amino acids are added to equivalent caloric amounts of fat emulsion or glucose, the latter combination results in a less negative nitrogen balance[6] (Figs. 2.3 and 2.5). In severely injured man, some investigators have failed to observe any reduction in nitrogen sparing with the infusion of large doses of soybean fat emulsions.[14] In similar patients, however, others have noted improvement in nitrogen sparing when fat is added to amino acids but the degree of sparing is not equivalent to an equal caloric amount of glucose.[6] It has been proposed that the beneficial effects of fat emulsion on nitrogen sparing are the result of glycerol, a three carbon, carbohydrate-like energy source, contained in the fat emulsion.[15] In view of the degree of nitrogen sparing observed in normal and injured man when used in combination with amino acids, it appears that fat emulsions are helpful in sparing nitrogen to a greater extent than can be attributed to its glycerol content alone,[6, 14] but it is important to note that with respect to nitrogen sparing glucose and amino acids are much more effective than fat, calorie for calorie.

Although there are no distinct differences in nitrogen balance when comparing low dose isosmotic administration of glucose and amino acids, there are clear advantages to infusing a medium dose combination of the two substrates. First, their effect is augmentative and the impact of

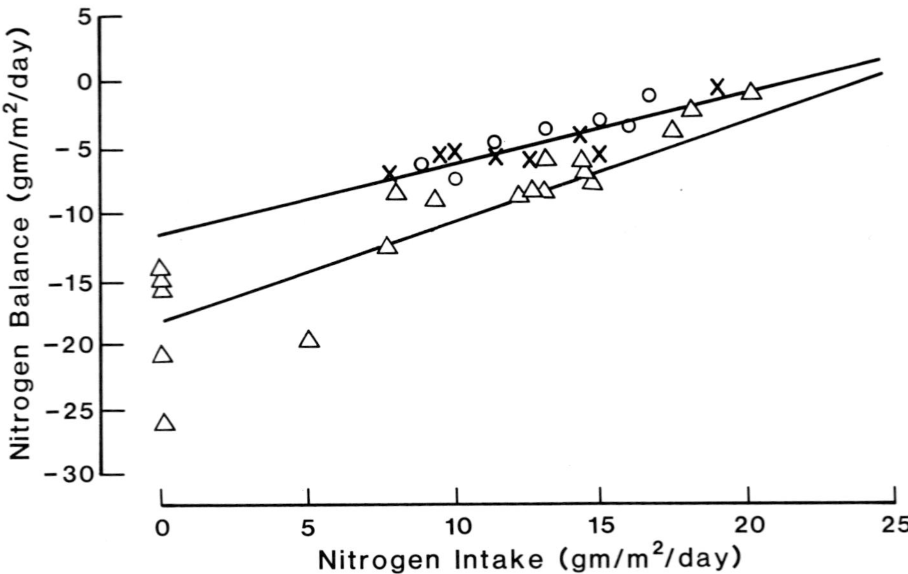

Figure 2.5. Nitrogen balance as a function of increasing caloric amounts of amino acids plus 28 or 56 g fat. △, amino acids without fat addition; ×, amino acids plus 28 g fat; ○, amino acids plus 56 g fat. Notice that there is no significant difference between 28 and 56 g fat therefore only one regression line has been drawn combining the two regimens.

calories is not limited when protein is provided. Second amino acids administered alone cause a constant rise in the blood urea nitrogen which is not observed when glucose is added. Third, altered liver and renal transport occur in critically ill patients who are given amino acids as their sole caloric source. The altered transport properties may be restored to normal by glucose addition. An appropriate combination which provides maximal nitrogen sparing per gram nutrient administered while maintaining optimal hepatic, renal, and cardiac function consists of 30 g glucose plus 5 g amino nitrogen per liter of fluid (600 cc Dextrose 5% in water plus 400 cc FreAmine II). This solution is given at a rate to satisfy normal fluid requirements of the traumatized or postoperative patient. Fat emulsion (Intralipid) given in 500 cc amounts once or twice a day provides additional calories but should not be used as a substitute for either glucose or amino acids.

Since these solutions may be administered by peripheral vein and since alterations in infusion rate and even abrupt cessation of the infusion can be accomplished without untoward effects so that blood, antibiotics, and other medications can be given, these infusates are an ideal means of preserving normal metabolic function of vital organs while limiting nitrogen loss in immediately post-traumatic, postoperative, and unstable critically ill patients. Unfortunately, it is generally not possible to achieve a positive nitrogen balance with isosmotic solutions since the amount of calories required would necessitate excessive fluid administration. Should illness be protracted and oral alimentation not a reality, positive nitrogen balance is achieved by administration of hyperosmotic solutions (hyper-alimentation).

Central Parenteral or Hyperosmotic Intravenous Nutrition

Hyperosmotic intravenous solutions which are capable of providing enough nitrogen and calories in an acceptable volume are made up of equivalent amounts of an 8.5% amino acid solution (FreAmine II) and 50% Dextrose and water thereby providing approximately one kcal/cc solution. Electrolytes and twice the daily requirement of vitamins are added (Table 2.3). In addition, essential fatty acids are provided by the administration of 500 cc of fat emulsion two to three times weekly. Trace elements and other essential serum components are given by the administration of fresh frozen plasma two to four times weekly. With this hyperosmotic glucose amino acid solution up to 4000 kcal/day may be infused and a positive nitrogen balance can be established.

Because the hyperalimentation solution is hyperosmotic, it must be administered through a central venous line and its rate of administration must be rigidly controlled. The central venous line must be placed and maintained using assiduous sterile technique for if not infection will invariably follow. The skin over the puncture site is initially defatted with ether and then cleansed with an iodophor. The intravenous line is placed into the superior vena cava either by subclavian or internal jugular puncture. The area is dressed sterilly and an antibiotic ointment placed over the catheter entrance site. On alternate days, the dressing is changed and a new sterile dressing, iodophor prep and antibiotic ointment applied. A millipore filter is placed in line and the filter and intravenous tubing changed and cultured every 24 hours. No medications, blood, or other fluids should be administered through the hyperalimentation line nor should central venous pressure measurements be made utilizing the catheter through which the hyperalimentation solution is being administered. The fluid should be administered initially at low rates (50 cc/hr) until tolerance has been achieved (blood glucose remains below 200 mg%) after which the rate of infusion may be gradually increased until the

Table 2.3
Composition of hyperalimentation solution

FreAmine II (8.5%)	500 cc
$D_{50}W$	500 cc
NaCl	40–50 mEq
KCl	20–40 mEq
K_2HPO_4	10 mEq
Ca gluconate	10 mEq
$MgSO_4$	8 mEq
Vitamin B_{12}*	1000 μg
Folate*	0.5 mg
Vitamin K*	5 mg
Vitamin C*	500 mg
MVI* (Multiple vitamin infusion)	1 amp

* May be added once per 24 hours.

proper caloric load is achieved. Usually 3 to 4 liters are given daily, thus providing the patient with 3000 to 4000 kcal/24 hours. The urine must be monitored for sugar every 4 hours and, when present, the infusion rate either reduced or insulin administered. Plasma osmolality and Na, K, Cl, CO_2, BUN, Cr, Ca, PO_4, and glucose should also be monitored on a frequent periodic basis (initially, daily). Magnesium levels should be monitored regularly but somewhat less frequently. When discontinuing the infusion, the rate should be gradually tapered over a 24 to 36 hour period.

Complications are not infrequent and can be life threatening. Placement of the central venous catheter has resulted in pneumothorax, hemothorax, hydrothorax, brachial plexus injury, arterial injury, venous thrombosis, and embolism. Because of the nature of the solution infused and the central venous location of the catheter, infectious complications have been reported to be between 10 and 30%. *Candida albicans* is particularly common. *Candida* overgrowth can be effectively reduced by the daily prophylactic installation of 1 mg Amphotericin B into the catheter. Infections of the central line result in septicemia, metastatic abscesses and acute bacterial endocarditis emphasizing the need for rigid sterile technique in caring for the line.

Numerous metabolic complications may occur and must be recognized and immediately corrected if patient survival is to be maximal[16] (Table 2.4). Alterations in glucose metabolism may result in hyperglycemia, glycosuria with an osmotic diuresis and in severe cases hyperosmolar

Table 2.4
Metabolic complications of central venous hyperalimentation

Glucose metabolism
  Hyperglycemia
    1. Osmotic diuresis
    2. Hyperosmolar nonketotic diabetic coma
  Postinfusion hypoglycemia
Amino acid metabolism
  Hyperchloremic metabolic acidosis
  Hyperammoniemia
  Prerenal azotemia
Fat metabolism
  Essential fatty acid deficiencies
  Lipemic serum
  Febrile response to infusate
Electrolytes
  Hypophosphatemia
  Hyper and hyponatremia
  Hyper and hypokalemia
  Hypomagnesemia
  Hyper- and hypocalcemia
Miscellaneous
  Fatty infiltration of the liver
  Cholestatic jaundice
  Abnormal liver chemistries
  Hyper- and hypovitaminosis
  Anemia

     TRAUMATIC INJURIES OF THE GENITOURINARY SYSTEM

nonketotic dehydration and coma. Early recognition of hyperglycemia and its treatment by reducing the rate of infusion and/or insulin administration correct these complications. Patients with nonketotic hyperosmolar coma characteristically have blood sugars above 500 mg% and must be treated aggressively, often with large doses of insulin and fluid. Ketoacidosis in diabetic patients given inadequate insulin for the additional carbohydrate load and postinfusion hypoglycemia resulting from rapid withdrawal of glucose in the face of persistently elevated endogenous insulin levels may also occur and are treated by increasing insulin and glucose infusion, respectively.

Alterations in amino acid metabolism may result in hyperchloremic metabolic acidosis, plasma amino acid imbalances, hyperammoniemia and elevated blood urea nitrogen levels. When these occur, alterations in the content of the infusate or rate of infusion must be made. Hypophosphatemia and hyper- and hypocalcemia are corrected by addition or removal to the infusate of the appropriate inorganic ion. Vitamin deficiencies, essential fatty acid deficiencies, trace mineral deficiencies, abnormal plasma potassium, sodium, and magnesium levels have all been reported and are corrected by appropriate addition or removal of the particular substance. Trace minerals and essential fatty acid deficiencies are not encountered when fresh frozen plasma and fat emulsions are administered as described above. Finally alterations in liver enzymes, cholestatic jaundice and fatty infiltration of the liver complicate long term administration.

Intravenous Nutrition and Renal Failure

There is some evidence to indicate that seriously ill patients who sustain acute renal failure may be successfully managed by providing them with intravenous hyperosmotic glucose and essential amino acid solutions (hyperalimentation). When such solutions are administered to acute renal failure patients, a more rapid recovery of the renal dysfunction with a less rapid rise in the BUN during the period of acute renal failure is observed when such patients are compared to patients treated conservatively with lesser amounts of glucose.[17] Patients with renal failure require at least twice the amount of essential amino acids per day as do normal individuals but the ideal amount and combination of amino acids has yet to be defined.

REFERENCES

1. Passmore, R. Recommended intakes of nutrients for the United Kingdom. *Reports on Public Health and Medical Subjects*, No. 120:34 London, Her Majesty's Stationary Office, 1969.
2. Wilmore, D. W., Long, J. M., Mason, A. D. Jr., et al. Catecholamines: mediator of the hypermetabolic response to thermal injury. *Ann. Surg. 180:*653, 1974.
3. Kinney, J. M. The metabolic response to injury. In *Nutritional Aspects of Care in the Critically Ill.* Edited by J. R. Richards and J. M. Kinney. Churchill Livingstone, London, 1977.
4. Long, C. L., Spencer, J. L., Kinney, J. M., et al. Carbohydrate metabolism in normal man and effect of glucose infusion. *J. Appl. Physiol. 31:*102, 1971.

5. Wilmore, D. W., Mason, A. D., Jr., and Pruitt, B. A., Jr. Insulin response to glucose in hypermetabolic burn patients. *Ann. Surg. 183:*314, 1976.
6. McDougal, W. S., Wilmore, D. W. and Pruitt, B. A., Jr. Effect of near isosmotic intravenous nutrient infusions on nitrogen balance in critically ill injured patients. *Surg. Gynecol. Obstet. 145:*408, 1977.
7. Steiger, E., Daly, J. M., Allen, J. R., et al. Postoperative intravenous nutrition: effects on body weight, protein regeneration, wound healing and liver morphology. *Surgery* 73: 686, 1973.
8. Law, D. K., Dudreic, S. J., and Abdou, N. I. Immunocompetence of patients with protein-calorie malnutrition: the effects of nutritional repletion. *Ann. Intern. Med. 79:* 545, 1973.
9. McDougal, W. S., Wilmore, D. W. and Pruitt, B. A. Jr. Glucose dependent hepatic membrane transport in nonbacteremic and bacteremic thermally injured patients. *J. Surg. Res. 22:*697, 1977.
10. Montemurro, D. G. and Stevenson, J. A. Survival and body composition of normal and hypothalamic obese rats in acute starvation. *Am. J. Physiol. 198:* 757, 1960.
11. Wolfe, B. M., Culebras, J. M., Sim, A. J. W., et al. Substrate interaction in intravenous feeding. Comparative effects of carbohydrate and fat on amino acid utilization in fasting man. *Ann. Surg. 186:*518, 1977.
12. Calloway, D. H., Spector, H. Nitrogen balance as related to calorie and protein intake in active young men. *Am. J. Clin. Nutr. 2:*405, 1954.
13. Blackburn, G. L., Flatt, J. P., Clowes, G. G. A., et al. Protein sparing therapy during periods of starvation with sepsis or trauma. *Ann Surg. 177:*588, 1973.
14. Long, J. M., Wilmore, D. W., Mason, A. D. Jr., et al. Effect of carbohydrate and fat intake on nitrogen excretion during total intravenous feeding. *Ann. Surg. 185:*4417, 1977.
15. Brennan, M. F., Fitzpatrick, G. F., Cohen, K. H., et al. Glycerol: major contributor to the short term protein sparing effect of fat emulsions in normal man. *Ann Surg. 182:* 386, 1975.
16. Dudrick, S. J., MacFadyen, B. V., VanBuren, C. T., et al. Parenteral hyperalimentation. Metabolic problems and solutions. *Ann. Surg. 176:*259, 1972.
17. Abel, R. M., Beck, C. H., Jr., Abbott, W. M., et al: Improved survival from acute renal failure after treatment with intravenous essential L-amino acids and glucose. *N. Engl. J. Med. 288:*695, 1973.

 TRAUMATIC INJURIES OF THE GENITOURINARY SYSTEM

3

Traumatic Injuries of the External Genitalia

Proper management of the genital area following traumatic injuries not only requires a fundamental knowledge of urologic and plastic surgery principles but poses unique problems in patient management. Postinjury, many patients experience fear over the possible loss of sexual potency and reproductive ability. Early counseling and supportive discussions about what can be accomplished cosmetically and functionally are critical if behavioral problems are to be minimized during the reconstructive and postreconstructive periods. In addition to psychological problems which invariably accompany these injuries, the composition of the genital tissues poses special problems in surgical management. The skin has a very thin dermis beneath which lies a layer of loose areolar tissue. These characteristics result in marked edema when the tissue is traumatized, poor capacity of sutures to hold the tissues together when they are placed under tension, and extensive hematoma formation when the blood vessels beneath the skin are ruptured. There are also unique aspects of care which must be considered in the postoperative period. Erections in the immediate postsurgical period may result in bleeding and tension on the suture line. Moreover, the need to divert urine and feces away from healing wounds if their proximity will result in persistent contamination of the surgical repair must be considered. Initial evaluation of the external genitalia should include an appraisal of: 1) the perineal soft tissue and cutaneous loss, 2) the competence of the urinary and rectal sphincters, and 3) the integrity of the urethra and rectosigmoid colon.

AVULSION OF THE GENITAL SKIN

Extensive loss of the penile and/or scrotal skin is often the result of a degloving type injury. This injury occurs when the loose skin is caught with the clothing in a device which tears both from the patient. A moving belt on farm machinery is often the cause. Separation of the tissue occurs

39

in the loose areolar layer which is superficial to Buck's fascia in the penis
and immediately beneath the dartos muscle in the scrotum. The deeper
tissues including corpora, urethea, and testes are usually unharmed. The
avulsion characteristically involves the circumference of the shaft of the
penis from penile scrotal junction to corona. Scrotal involvement, however, does not characteristically result in the loss of the entire scrotal
covering.

Immediate repair is essential for delays will result in cicatrix formation,
development of contractures, and subsequent genital deformity. The
wounds should be thoroughly cleaned, foreign materials sought and
removed, nonviable tissue excised, and the integrity of the urethra and
testes confirmed.

Small noncircumferential defects in the penile skin may be closed
primarily after freshening the edges, provided there is no tension on the
suture line. When closure cannot be accomplished without tension, either
a full thickness graft taken from the foreskin in the uncircumcised or a
split thickness graft is employed. In contrast, circumferential penile shaft
skin losses require more aggressive debridement. All proximal viable
tissue is preserved; however, the skin distal to the defect irrespective of its
viability should be removed 2 to 3 mm proximal to the corona. Retention
of the distal tissue will result in the development of brawny edema due to
the interruption of lymphatic drainage (Fig. 3.1). The edema persists for

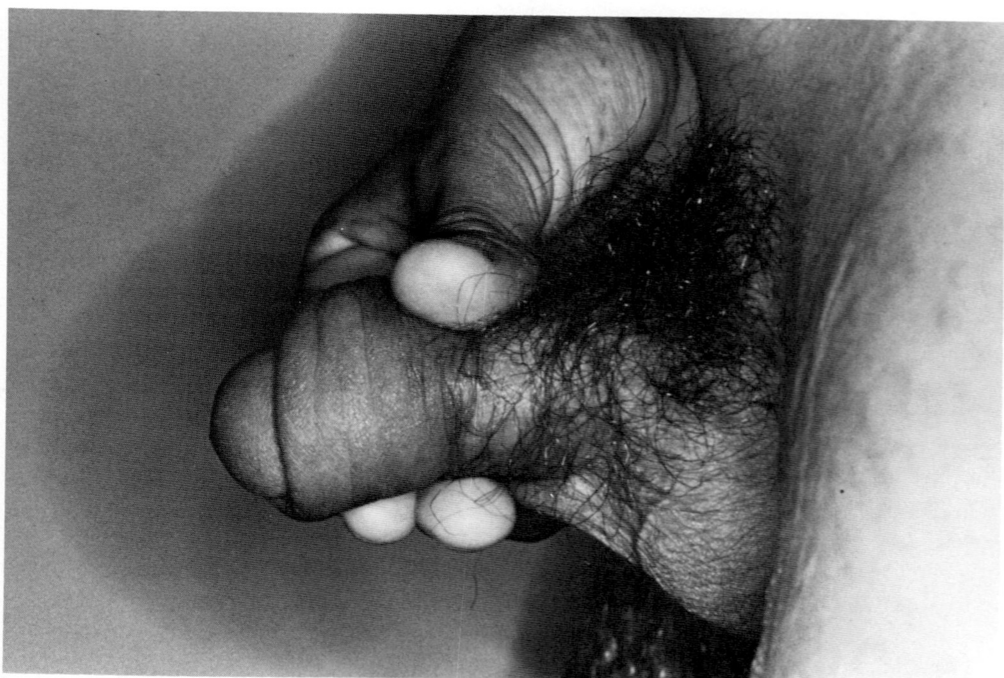

Figure 3.1. Brawny edema of the distal penile skin in a patient who had
sustained a circumferential penile wound and in whom the distal tissue was not
excised but rather used to resurface the injury.

    TRAUMATIC INJURIES OF THE GENITOURINARY SYSTEM

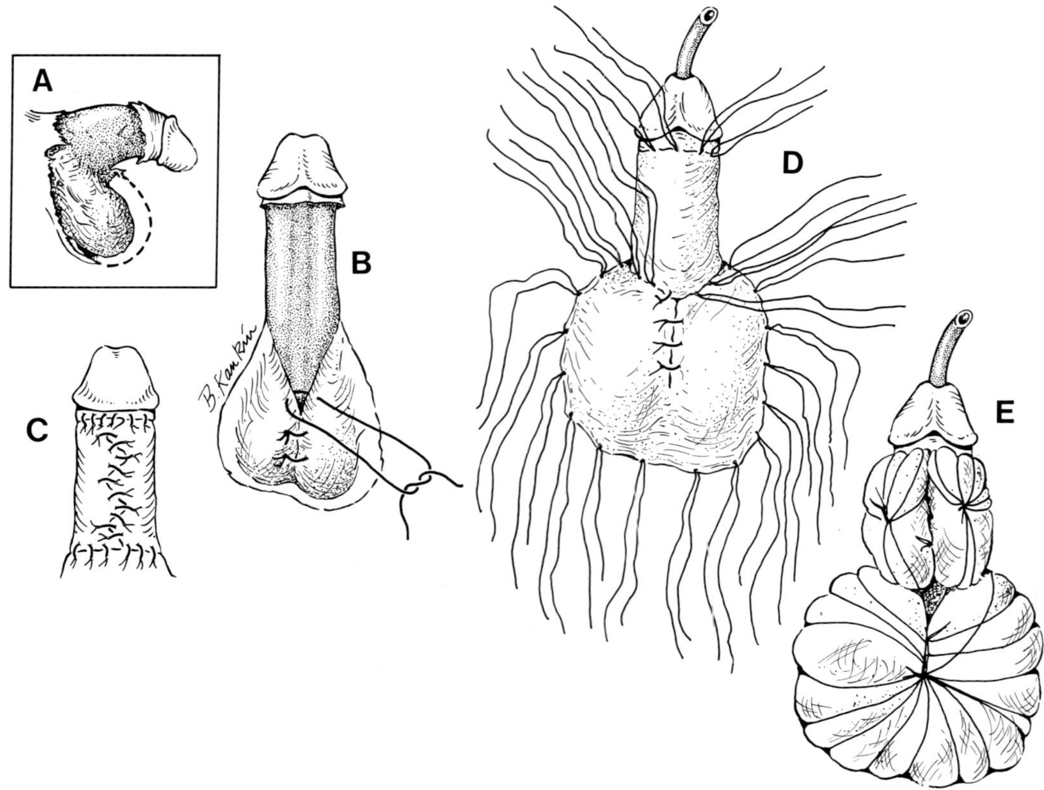

Figure 3.2. Avulsion injury. *A*, the injury which involves a circumferential skin loss from the penis and an extensive scrotal defect is illustrated. *B*, the skin on the distal shaft is removed. A margin of several millimeters of skin is left adjacent to the corona to which the skin graft will be sewn. The margins of the scrotal defect are debrided and the internal spermatic fascia overlying the testes is sutured together in the midline. *C*, the penile shaft is grafted with split thickness skin. The interdigitating seam is placed on the dorsum of the shaft. *D*, split thickness graft is applied over the scrotal defect and tailored to cover the testes. The sutures used to sew the margin of the graft in place are left long. *E*, the grafts are stented using cotton wadding which is held in place by tying the sutures at the margin over the wadding.

months to years, making both the appearance and function of the part unsatisfactory to most patients.

The defects created by extensive losses of the penile and scrotal skin are covered with thick split thickness graft and stented. The stent is formed from cotton wadding soaked in glycerol and is held in place by leaving the sutures at the margin of the graft long and tying them over the wadding. The grafts are taken at a thickness of 0.016 to 0.018 inches in the adult. The epithelium in children is not as thick as it is in the adult and, therefore, in the young, the graft is taken at a thickness of 0.010 to 0.014 inches. Circumferential wounds of the penis are covered by a single sheet of graft sewn in place utilizing the technique of an interdigitating seam located on the dorsum of the penis (Fig. 3.2). The graft is stented for 4 to 7 days, a transurethral Foley placed, and the Foley taped to the abdomen so that the penis is maintained in the anatomic position. The interdigitating seam breaks the line of scar formation and the dorsal placement provides for a functional result should scar contracture occur, *i.e.* a slight dorsal curvature is functionally better tolerated than a ventral curvature.

All viable scrotal tissue should be preserved, for its elasticity will often allow for complete coverage of the defect without the necessity for skin grafts. The wound margins are freshened and brought together with interrupted 3-0 reabsorbable suture. Extensive losses of scrotal skin do not allow for primary closure and result in exposure of the testes. These structures must be covered in such a way as to assure that their temperature will remain a few degrees below core body temperature if fertility is to be preserved. There are two methods of accomplishing this purpose: split thickness skin coverage[1] and transferal to superficial subcutaneous thigh pockets.[2] If the testes are uninjured and have a good blood supply, they are sutured together in the midline, covered with split thickness graft and stented (Fig. 3.2). The stent may be removed in 4 to 7 days. A very acceptable cosmetic result is obtained, morbidity is minimized, and the thin covering results in reduced testicular temperature, thereby allowing spermatogenesis to proceed normally. If the viability of the testes is in doubt or their blood supply is marginal, each testis is implanted into the adjacent thigh. The perineal defect is closed with a split thickness skin graft and stented in place. The testes should be implanted in a superficial subcutaneous pouch so that their temperature is maintained below that of the body core temperature. The implantation should be carefully planned with the thought in mind that the skin immediately overlying the testes will be used for reconstructing the scrotum. They should be placed slightly posterior and at asymmetric levels to prevent trauma during ambulation. The scrotum is reconstructed at a later date using the thigh skin and subcutaneous tissue containing the testes as pedicle flaps (Fig. 3.3). Split thickness skin grafts will alow the patient to appreciate gross tactile sensation but generally do not provide for the finer sensations of pin prick, two point discrimination, pain and temperature.

PENILE GANGRENE

Traumatic gangrene of the penis may involve only the skin and subcutaneous tissue or it may affect the full thickness of the organ. It is the result of the placement of a constriction about the penis usually as a form of masturbation, as a means of maintaining an erection, or as a form of child abuse. Many objects have been used and include nuts, pieces of pipe, string, rubber bands, wire, condoms, and hair. The latter is commonly the constricting agent in cases where the gangrene is the result of child abuse. Initially, the constricting band impedes superficial venous return but does not prevent arterial inflow or deep venous outflow. Distal skin and subcutaneous edema and necrosis result. Unchecked, the edema progresses and impedes arterial inflow. When this occurs, gangrene of the

TRAUMATIC INJURIES OF THE GENITOURINARY SYSTEM

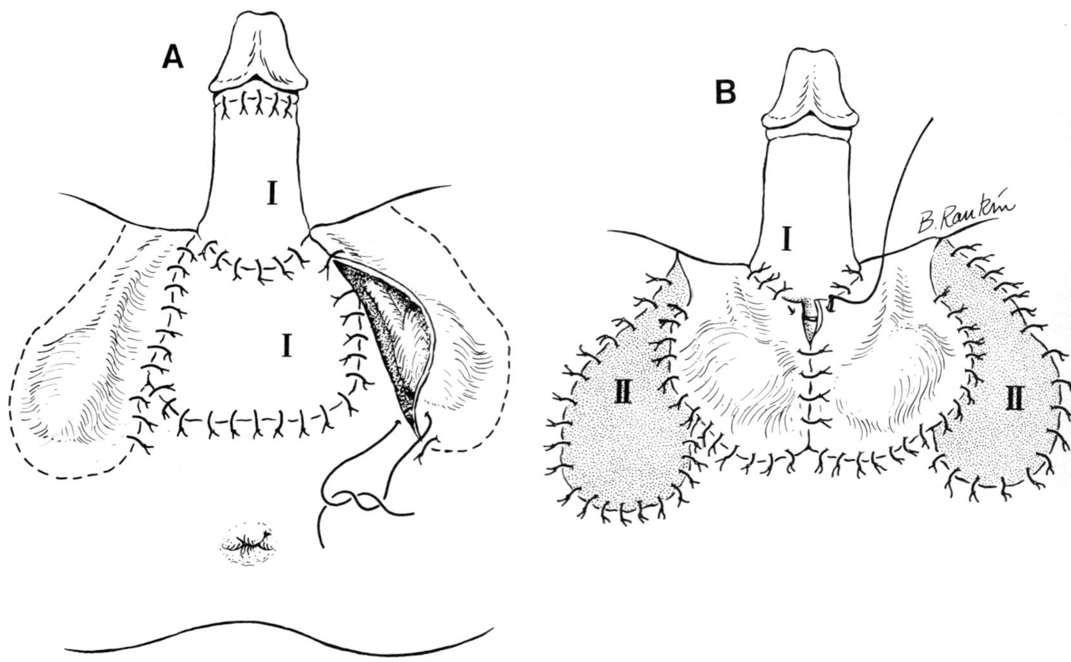

Figure 3.3. Implantation of the testes into the thighs with subsequent reconstruction of the scrotum from thigh pedicle flaps. *A*, the testes are implanted into superficial subcutaneous pockets on the posteriomedial aspect of the thighs. The denuded penile shaft and perineal defect are grafted with split thickness skin (*I*) and stented as described in Figure 3.2. *B*, after 1 to 2 months, the thigh pedicle flaps containing the testes are raised and rotated medially. The split thickness skin graft on the perineum is removed, and the pedicle grafts are sutured together in the midline and to the margins of the defect posteriorly and laterally. The wounds created on the medial aspect of the thighs are closed with split thickness skin grafts (*II*) and stented in place.

entire structure distal to the obstruction is imminent. Initially, the ability to void may be undisturbed; however, as the edema progresses, the patient may have considerable difficulty micturating. When these injuries are recognized early, before gangrene is present, metal bands may be cut and removed, or slipped off by threading a string through the band, wrapping the distal penis with the string after several puncture holes have been made in the distal skin to allow edema fluid to escape, and unwrapping the string from the proximal aspect of the band. Occasionally, the metal band cannot be cut nor can it be removed by the string technique. Under these circumstances, the penile skin and subcutaneous tissue should be surgically excised to the level of Buck's fascia from object to corona.[3] The object can then be slid off and the penile shaft grafted as described for avulsion injuries (Fig. 3.2). String, wire, rubber bands and hair may be very difficult to find once edema has become significant. These objects tend to become buried and, if they cannot be appreciated, the penis

EXTERNAL GENITALIA INJURIES

should be anesthetized and a longitudinal slit should be made, beginning in the normal skin and extending onto the area of edema. This will result in severance of the band.

After the constricting agent is removed, an assessment of the extent of necrosis must be made. If the gangrene extends to the deep tissues, a suprapubic cystostomy should be placed and the lesion should be treated with twice daily applications of a topical antimicrobial preceded by thorough cleansing with an iodophor. Mafenide acetate and silver sulfadiazine are both acceptable topical antimicrobials; however, mafenide acetate is preferred due to its better penetrability of the eschar. This therapy is continued until demarkation is unequivocally established. The gangrenous area is removed with an attempt to preserve as much penile length as possible. The procedure is identical too a standard partial penectomy.

AMPUTATION OF THE PENIS WITH RETENTION OF THE TRANSECTED PART

Amputation of the penis may be a result of a self-inflicted injury, an act of violence to the individual, a blast injury, or other mechanical trauma. Massive bleeding and shock are common sequelae. Hemostasis should be achieved by compression and not by indiscriminate ligation of bleeding vessels until blood pressure is restored to normal. This is important in order to assure the best possible chance for a successful microvascular repair. The amputated part is placed in iced Ringer's lactate containing penicillin and streptomycin. The dorsalis penis and profunda arteries and corpora cavernosa are flushed with cold heparinized saline until the venous effluent is clear. If the transection has occurred distal to the penile scrotal junction, a tourniquet may be applied to the proximal retained portion to achieve hemostasis. The proximal arteries and veins are identified, cannulated with polyethylene catheters, and flushed with heparinized saline. When brisk arterial bleeding is obtained, the vessels are occluded with noncrushing microvascular clips. The wound is irrigated and loose nonviable tissue removed. A suprapubic cystostomy or perineal urethrostomy is performed, the former being preferred since it may be accomplished without manipulation of the proximal penile stump. A Foley catheter is placed through the urethra of the severed part and thence through the proximal urethra into the bladder. This serves to align the structures to be sutured (Fig. 3.4). The urethra is the first structure to be anastomosed and is sutured together in an oblique manner with 4-0 atraumatic chromic suture. The corpora cavernosae are next sutured together with interrupted 5-0 Proline. These two structures must be sutured together first for they provide the necessary stability required for the subsequent microvascular anastomosis. It should be noted that some surgeons prefer to anastomose the profunda arteries in which case this must be accomplished following the urethral anastomosis and prior to the corpora anastomosis. These arteries are often impossible to find in the severed part and are not critical to an acceptable result. Using the operative microscope, the deep dorsal and superficial dorsal veins are each anastomosed with 9 or 10-0 nylon suture. Usually only one of the two veins can be found in which case one anastomosis is generally adequate. Attention is then turned to the two dorsal arteries which are sutured together with interrupted 10-0 nylon. The two dorsal nerves are identified and reapproximated with 10-0 nylon. The penis and glans should immediately "pink up" after release of the microsvascular clamps. Bleeding points from the severed edges may now be individually ligated. When adequate hemostasis has been achieved, Buck's fascia is loosely sutured together with 5-0 Proline. The skin is loosely brought together

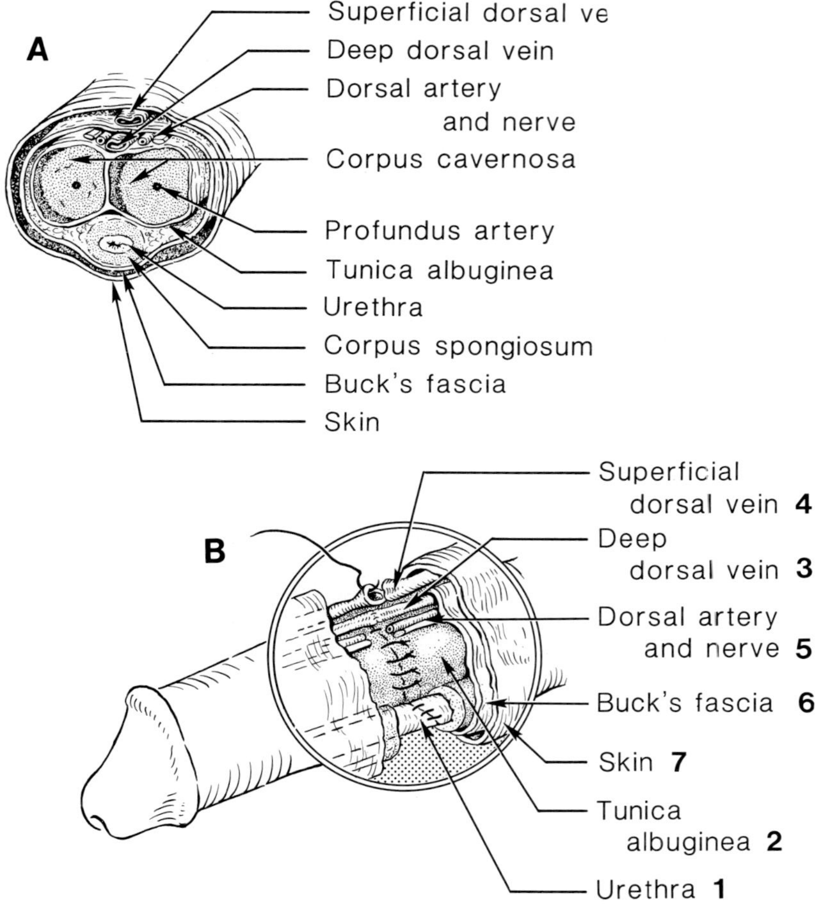

Figure 3.4. Microvascular repair of the amputated penis. *A*, cross sectional anatomy of the penile shaft. *B*, the urethra has been repaired in an oblique fashion over a stenting catheter (*1*) and the tunica albuginea of the corpora cavernosa have been reapproximated (*2*). Using a microvascular technique, the deep dorsal vein has been repaired (*3*) and the superficial dorsal vein is being reanastomosed (*4*). The deep dorsal arteries and nerves (*5*) are subsequently reapproximated. Finally, Buck's fascia (*6*) and the skin (*7*) are loosely sutured together.

EXTERNAL GENITALIA INJURIES

with 4 or 5-0 nonreabsorbable suture. A bulky dressing is placed on the penis and it is taped to abdominal wall.[4, 5]

The use of anticoagulants in the postoperative period is controversial. Bleeding into the penis with large hematoma formation has been reported with the use of heparin. Urokinase and low molecular weight dextran have also been employed with some success.[4] Edema invariably occurs postoperatively but generally subsides by 2 to 3 weeks. Some superficial skin loss may occur which will require the application of split thickness skin as described in the section on avulsion injuries. Slight scarring and contracture of the corpora cavernosae at the level of the anastomosis is to be expected but has little consequence.[5] Sensation to light touch and pin prick returns by 3 months. The cosmetic and functional result is excellent, many patients reporting satisfactory erections and ejaculations. Successful microvascular replantations have been reported up to 18 hours post-injury. Complications include urethral strictures, urethral fistulae, distal skin necrosis, poor sensation, and inability to obtain or maintain erections.[6] These complications are much less common when the microvascular technique described above is employed than they are when the vessels are ligated and the amputated part is sutured in place using the urethra, corpora cavernosa, Buck's fascia, and skin.[7] Indeed, skin necrosis is so common with the latter method that it has been suggested that the penile skin should be removed from the severed part. Following the anastomosis, the penis is buried in the scrotum (Fig. 3.5). The shaft is released at a later date.[8]

AMPUTATION OF THE PENIS WITH LOSS OF THE TRANSECTED PART

This injury occurs as a result of amputation for malignancy, gun shot wounds, blast injuries, mechanical trauma and self-inflicted injury. Loss of the scrotum may often co-exist. The wounds should be debrided and

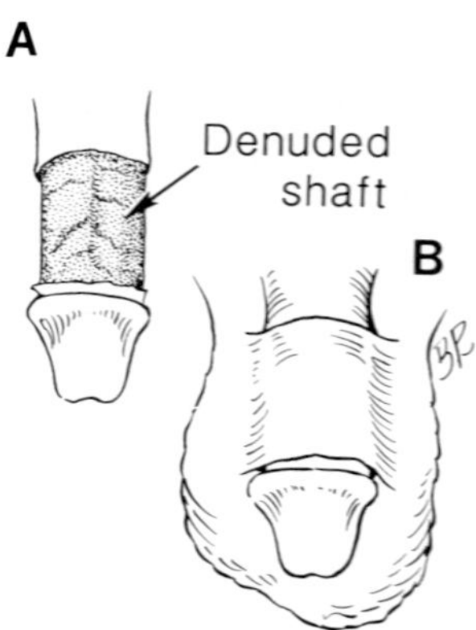

Figure 3.5.   Scrotal flap technique for covering a denuded penile shaft. The denuded penile shaft, *A*, is placed beneath a scrotal flap, *B*. The glans is exposed.

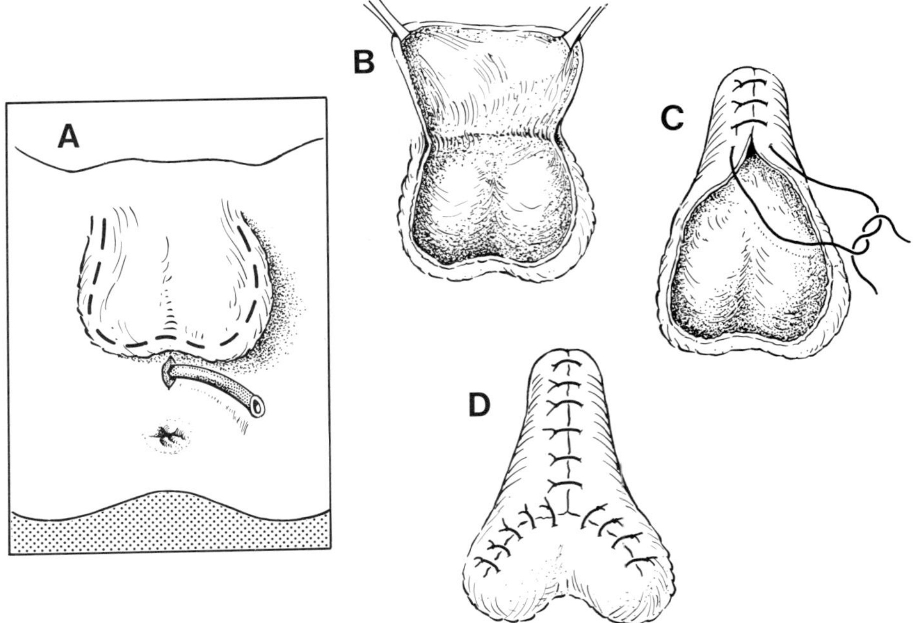

Figure 3.6. Reconstruction of the penis from scrotal tissues. *A*, the penis has been amputated and a perineal urethrostomy has been created. These wounds have been allowed to heal for several months. The incision to be made in the scrotum is outlined. *B*, a scrotal flap is raised with meticulous attention to hemostasis. *C*, the lateral margins of the scrotal flap are sutured together to create a cylinder. *D*, the scrotal defect is closed.

the defect closed either primarily or with split thickness skin (the former is preferred since it makes subsequent surgery less complicated). The reconstructive procedures are begun 1 to 3 months postinjury to allow for adequate healing of the perineal wounds.

When the scrotum is present, a nonfunctional, purely cosmetic appendage may be created from the scrotal tissues (Fig. 3.6). This structure over the long term is prone to shrinkage, atrophy, and deformity. In an attempt to prevent these complications, one testis and its cord have been translocated into the scrotal appendage. Initial results are encouraging.[9] Voiding is performed through a perineal urethrostomy.

A more functional structure may be created by constructing the penis from a tubed pedicle graft as originally described by Gilles and Harrison[10] and subsequently modified by others (Fig. 3.7). The structure allows the patient to void in the standing position, is cosmetically acceptable, and may be used for coitus, provided cartilage or a silastic rod has been implanted in it. The cartilage or silastic prosthesis is implanted in either side of the pedicle tube in the fatty tissue between the skin and neourethra 3 to 4 months following final attachment of the pedicle. The proximal part of the rigid stent is anchored to the corpora bodies. The prosthesis should extend along the entire length of the pedicle for if it falls short, a

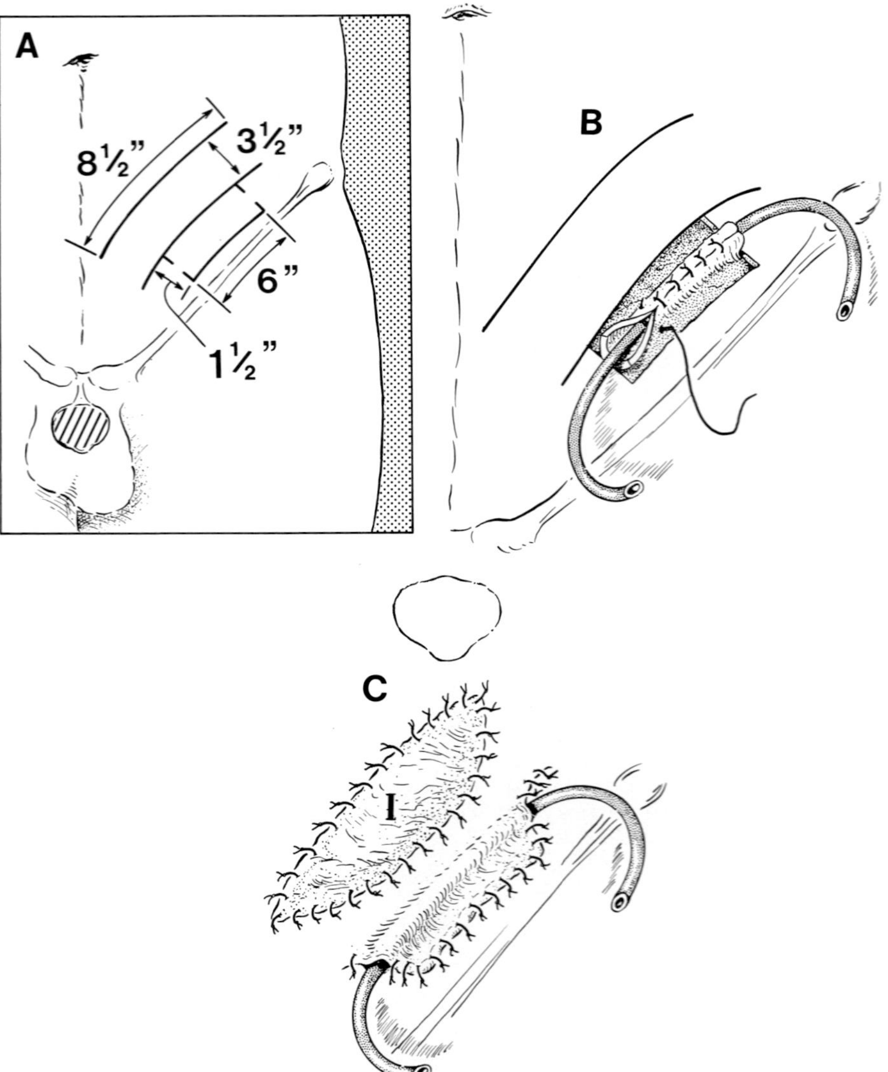

Figure 3.7. Reconstruction of the penis utilizing a tubed pedicle graft. *A*, the lines of incision, their position, and their dimensions are illustrated. *B*, a neourethra is constructed by raising two thin flaps and suturing the margins together with fine interrupted chromic over a stenting catheter so that the skin lies adjacent to the catheter. Care must be taken not to undermine the central one-half inch strip of skin for the neourethra is dependent upon this attachment for its blood supply. *C*, the bipedicle flap is mobilized, placed over the neourethra, and sutured laterally to the margin of the wound. Excellent hemostasis must be obtained and the pedicle must not be placed under tension. The medial defect is covered with a split-thickness skin graft (*I*) which may be stented in place. Frequent postoperative checks are necessary to prevent hematoma formation. *D*, after 3 to 4 weeks, the bipedicle graft is tubed to include the neourethra. The skin edges of the pedicle tube must be brought together on the posterior surface without tension. Excision of fat may be required at this stage to achieve a tension-free suture line. The defect created beneath the tube is covered with a split thickness skin graft (*II*). After several weeks, the stenting catheter may be removed, the neourethra flushed with saline, and a new catheter placed. A suprapubic cystostomy for urinary diversion is placed lateral to the midline on the contralateral side. *E*, after 1 to 3 months, an incision is made across one-half of the cephalad end of the pedicle. One week later the cephalad end is completely transected and the pedicle

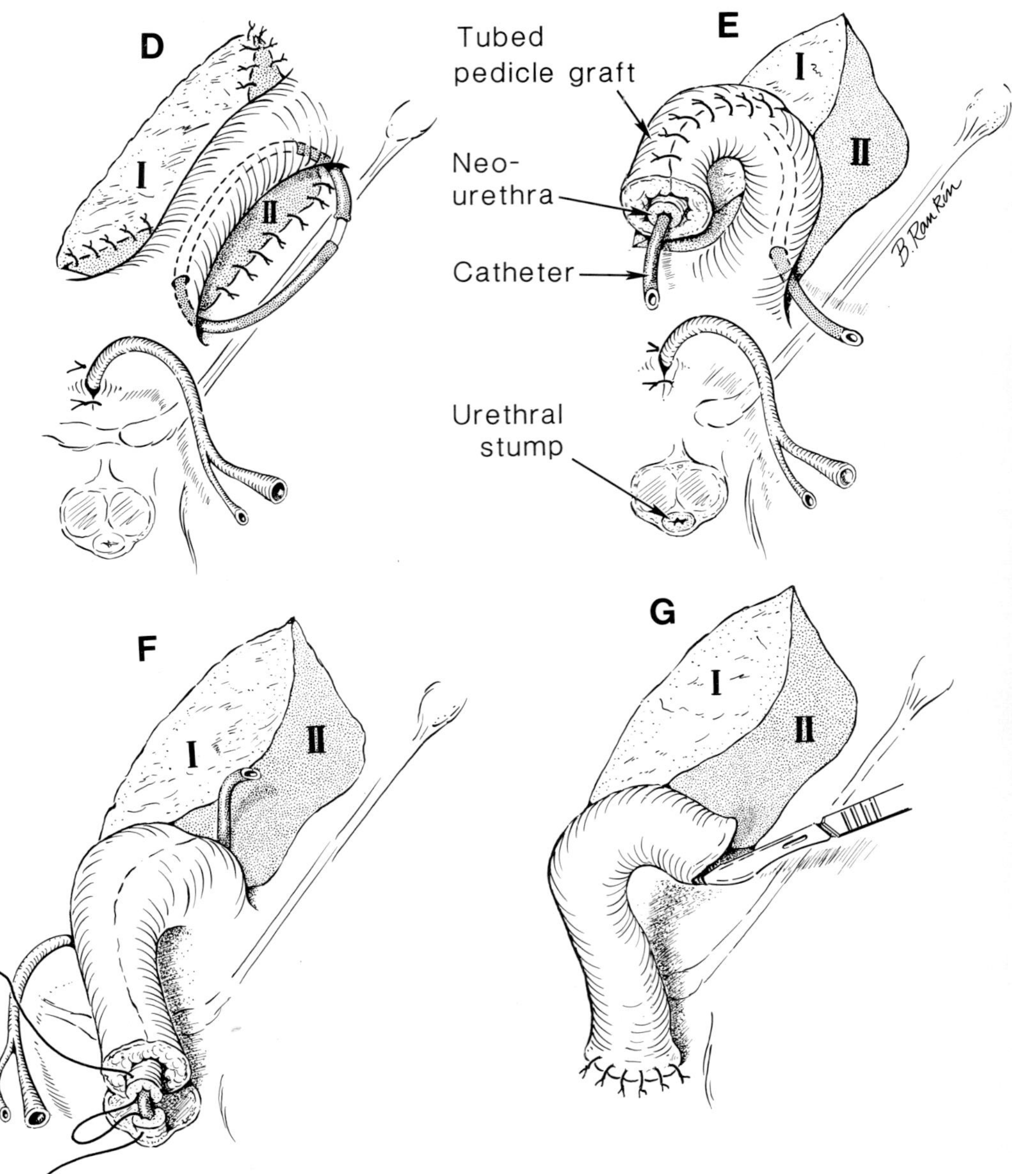

is rotated to the area of the urethral stump. Care must be taken not to kink or twist the base of the pedicle which remains attached to the abdominal wall for the viability of the pedicle is dependent upon the blood supply received through this portion of the graft. Supportive dressings may be required to assure a gentle curve. If the pedicle does not lay as desired and more length is required, two parallel incisions made at the base which extend toward the pubis will lengthen the graft. *F*, the neourethra is sutured in an oblique fashion to the urethral stump over a stenting catheter with fine interrupted chromic. The pedicle tube is sutured to a broad based defect made in the skin of the perineum. *G*, one to 2 months later, the abdominal attachment is severed. This may also be delayed by making an incision across one-half of the attachment followed 1 week later by complete transection. The skin margins on the end of the pedicle tube are sutured to the skin margins of the neourethra. Tip reconstruction, meatoplasty and implantation of cartilage or silastic prostheses are performed 3 to 6 months later after the vascular supply to the pedicle has become well established (adapted from Evans, 1963).

floppy end will result which will make intromission difficult. Complications of the reconstructive procedure include tissue slough, strictures, and urethral fistulae.[11, 12] A modification has been described in which an epithelialized channel is created by suturing the pedicle so that the epithelium forms a tube on the inside. Split thickness graft covers the exterior surface. This allows the patient to place a silastic tube in the channel and thereby transform the flaccid organ to a rigid one at will.[13] If absent, the scrotum is reconstructed with thigh pedicle flaps as illustrated in Figure 3.3. Another method of penile reconstruction involves the use of gracilis myocutaneous flaps. A myocutaneous flap is constructed in the standard fashion on each thigh, care being taken to preserve the delicate blood supply to the gracilis muscle. A tunnel is fashioned from the medial aspect of the thighs to the midline immediately beneath the symphysis pubis. Each flap is passed through the tunnel and brought out the midline defect. The flaps are sutured together in the midline and the skin of the flaps at the base is sutured to the edges of the defect immediately beneath the symphysis. Each flap forms the lateral one-half of the shaft of the penis. The structure is made rigid with the use of implants as described above. The patient voids through a perineal urethrostomy.

FRACTURE OF THE PENIS

Fracture of the penis occurs as a result of a forcible tear in one or both cavernous bodies during an erection. The wall of the corpora in the flacid state is normally 2 mm thick; however, during an erection, it has a thickness of ¼ to ½ mm, thereby making it much more susceptible to injury. The tear occurs as a result of blunt trauma and is usually located in the distal third, central part, or, rarely, at the root of the penis.[14] The urethra is involved in 30% of the cases.[15] A urethral injury should be suspected when blood is present at the meatus. A cracking noise is heard at the moment of injury and is followed by rapid detumescence. Pain may be severe. The penis appears contorted, echymotic, and edematous.

Two forms of therapy have been advocated provided the urethra is uninjured: conservative and surgical. Conservative therapy involves application of ice packs to the area, elevation of the part, injection of enzymatic agents and subsequent hematoma evacuation if they become troublesome.[16] This management provides an acceptable result in 90% of patients so treated. Others suggest that the surgical approach affords better functional results with reduced morbidity.[17] The tear is usually longitudinal and is repaired with interrupted 3-0 Prolene suture. The hematoma is evacuated, the wound closed, a compression dressing applied, and antibiotics administered. Irrespective of the method of treatment, erections must be prevented during the healing period. This may be accomplished by the oral administration of stilbestrol. It should be noted that patients who have sustained a concomitant urethral injury require a surgical approach.[18] The corpora are repaired before the urethral injury is approached.

    TRAUMATIC INJURIES OF THE GENITOURINARY SYSTEM

TESTICULAR RUPTURE

Rupture of the testes occurs as a result of blunt or penetrating trauma. Following injury, a large intrascrotal hematoma develops. Occasionally, the hematoma follows the plane of Colles' and Scarpa's fascia and extends onto the anterior abdominal wall. These injuries require early surgical exploration. The necrotic tissue should be debrided, viable extruding seminiferous tubules returned to the testis and the tunica albuginea sutured together with interrupted 3-0 chromic. Rarely, a portion of the tunica albuginae is lost and the defect cannot be primarily reapproximated. It may be covered with a free graft of tunica vaginalis.

The necessity for early exploration and repair is apparent when the results of nonintervention are compared to early surgical therapy. Eighty percent of patients explored early and repaired maintain viable testes, whereas only 33% of patients treated conservatively are found to have viable testes on follow up examination.[19]

THE BURNED PERINEUM

Burns of the perineum are rarely isolated injuries but rather occur in patients who have sustained major total body surface area burns.[20] Although treatment must be integrated with the care of the patient as a whole, two general principles apply to perineal burns: 1) preservation of

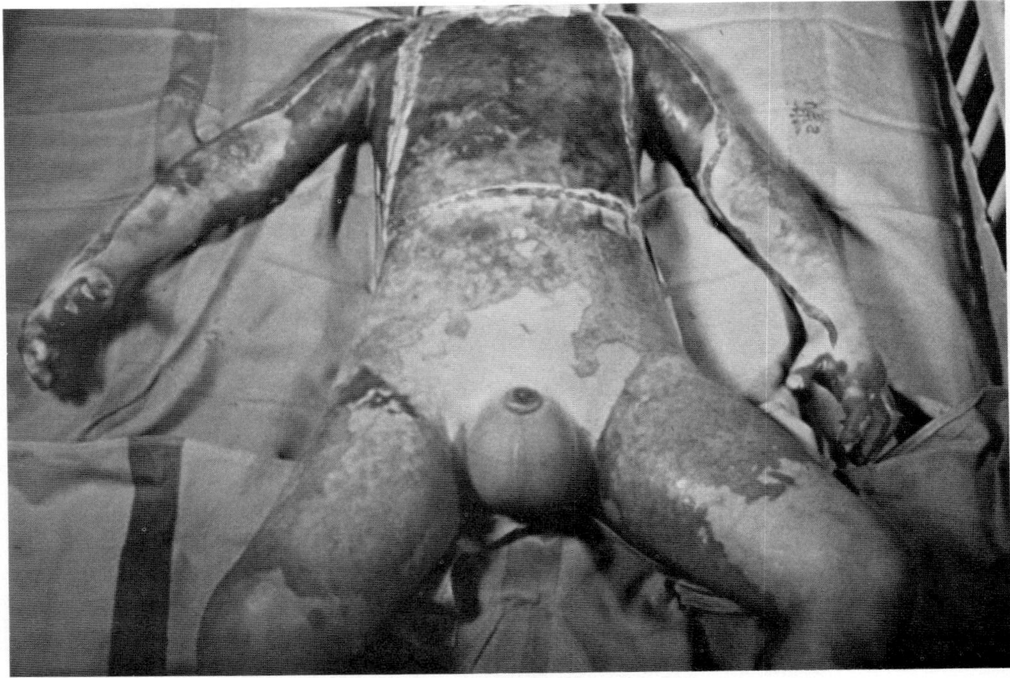

Figure 3.8.   Massive edema of the scrotum in a burn patient 48 hours postinjury.

as much tissue as possible is the goal, and, therefore, there is no place for radical debridement in these injuries, and 2) wound coverage should be obtained as rapidly as possible. Initial therapy of the perineal burn is dependent upon whether it is due to a thermal, chemical, or electric injury. All clothing is removed. Thermal injuries, if of limited extent, may be cooled (frost bite is rapidly rewarmed) and chemical injuries are copiously irrigated with water or saline. The use of neutralizing agents for chemical burns has no place in perineal injuries. Electric injuries are deceptive for a small area of skin injury may belie an extensive soft tissue necrosis below. In all types of injury, the loose tissue is removed and the hair overlying and adjacent to the area is shaved. The wound is gently washed with an iodophor and a topical antimicrobial is applied (mafenide acetate, silver sulfadiazine, or 0.5% silver nitrate soaks). Twice daily thereafter, the wound is washed with an iodophor and the antimicrobial reapplied. Mafenide acetate is preferred because of its broad spectrum coverage and its ability to penetrate beneath the eschar. With its use, however, staphylococci and fungi may emerge as a significant problem in the burn wound.

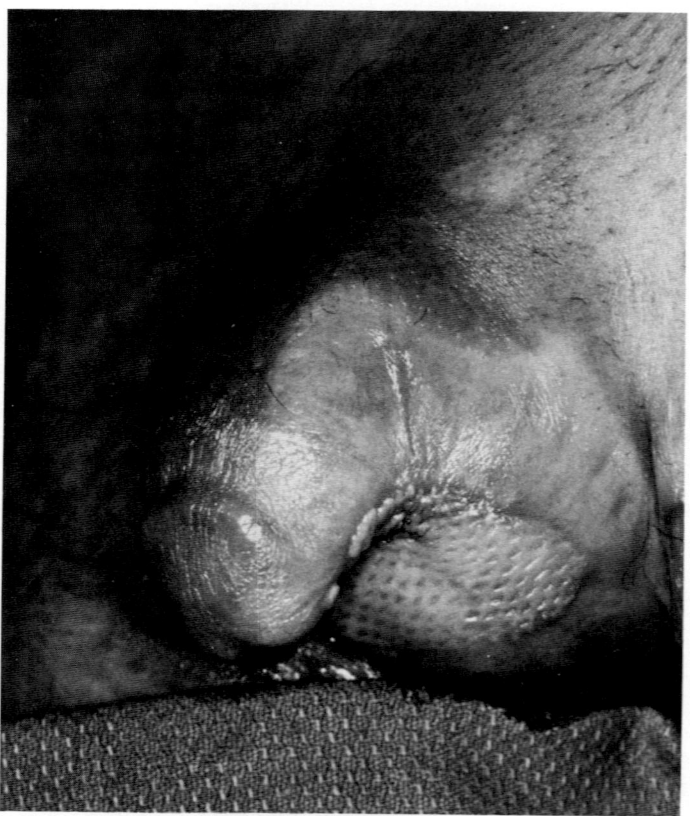

Figure 3.9. Deep second degree burns of the perineum often result in contracture formation and penile deformity as demonstrated in this patient.

TRAUMATIC INJURIES OF THE GENITOURINARY SYSTEM

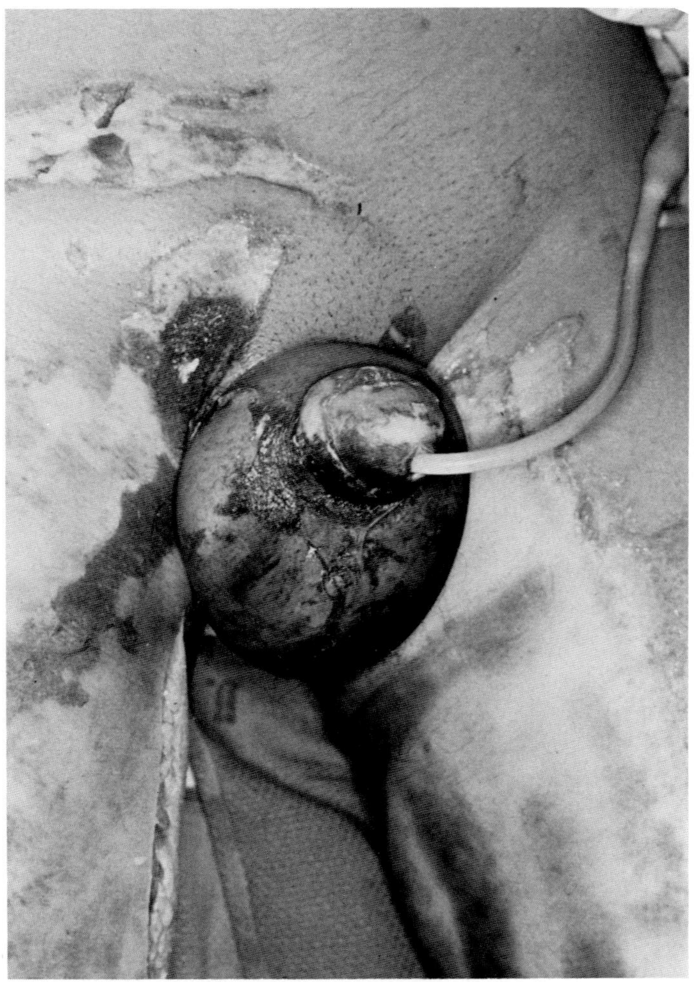

Figure 3.10.   A full thickness or third degree burn of the external genitalia.

Burns are classified according to the depth of injury as first, second, or third degree. A first degree injury involves only the epidermis, has an erythematous appearance, and is painful. First degree injuries of the perineum, particularly when accompanied by a large fluid resuscitation, often result in massive swelling of the genital tissues (Fig. 3.8). These injuries are treated by elevation and exposure (application of a topical antimicrobial is optional). The swelling subsides in 2 to 6 days postinjury and healing is complete by 6 to 10 days. Second degree or partial thickness injuries involve the epidermis and part of the dermis. They are red in appearance, may blister, are sensitive, and will spontaneously heal if burn wound sepsis does not supervene. These injuries are treated by twice daily iodophor washes and topical antimicrobial application. A urethral catheter is usually necessary early in the course but may be removed as healing commences. Healing is complete in 2 to 3 weeks. Contracture

EXTERNAL GENITALIA INJURIES   53

formation, particularly in deep second degree injuries, is a common sequelae in the ensueing months (Fig. 3.9). Third degree or full thickness injuries involve all of the epithelium, dermis, and deep dermal structures. They appear white to charred, are insensitive and will not heal (Fig. 3.10). These injuries must be grafted. Treatment involves twice daily iodophor washes followed by application of a topical antimicrobial and conservative debridement. Conservative debridement of the eschar involves the daily removal of loose and separating tissue. This process takes 2 to 3 weeks for complete eschar removal. Granulation tissue covers the defect and when it bleeds readily and is red in appearance, the wound is ready for the application of split thickness graft. If the granulation tissue is gray in appearance or does not bleed readily, it may be prepared by the application of wet dressings for several days, or it may be covered with homograft (cadaver skin) or xenograft (pig skin). The latter are removed at 5- to 7-day intervals until a healthy base of granulation tissue which will accept a split thickness graft, is formed. The shaft of the penis should

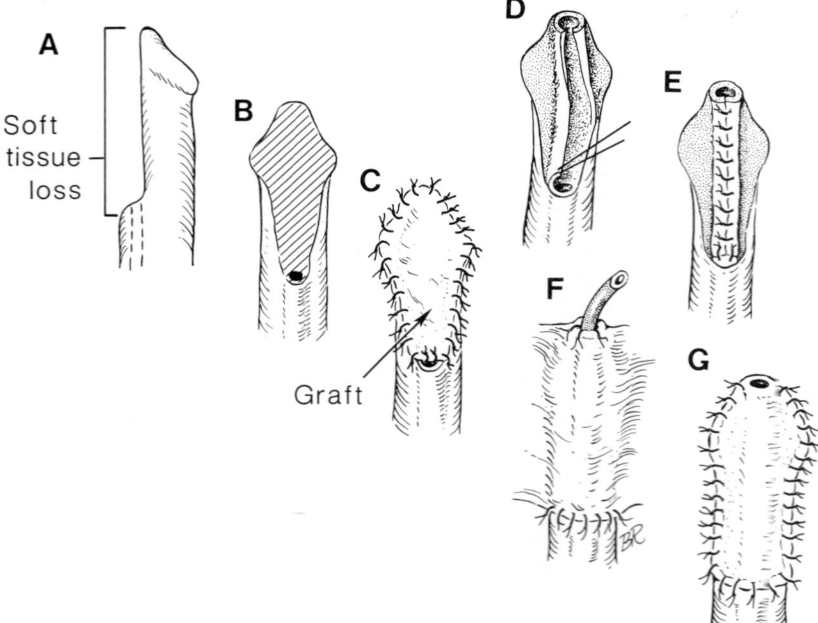

Figure 3.11. Repair of a penile soft tissue loss associated with a penile scrotal hypospadias. The injury viewed from the lateral aspect, *A*, and the ventral aspect, *B*, of the penis. *C*, a suprapubic cystostomy is placed and a full thickness skin graft taken from a non hair-bearing area is sutured over the defect and stented in place. *D*, after 4 to 6 weeks, the margins of the graft are raised being careful not to undermine the central strip of skin. *E*, a neourethra is constructed by suturing the margins together with fine interrupted chromic. The urethra is mobilized and sutured to the neourethra over a stenting catheter. *F*, the distal shaft is placed beneath a superficial abdominal flap. *G*, after 1 to 2 months, the flap may be severed from the abdominal wall and its margin sutured to the shaft of the penis. (A delayed technique is preferred. One side of the graft is transected and sutured to the penis. Several weeks later, the opposite side is severed.)

be grafted with sheet split thickness skin (0.16 to 0.18 inches thick) as depicted in Figure 3.2 and stented for 4 to 6 days. The scrotum may be grafted with either sheet or meshed graft. The latter is meshed 1½ to 1 and has the advantage of allowing drainage through the interstices of the graft. It provides a cover which looks very much like scrotal skin when healing is complete.

Urethral catheters are routinely employed in those with either perineal or large total body surface burns. They should be removed as early as possible and replaced only during periods of perineal grafting. Indeed, patients who have sustained full thickness burns to the ventrum of the penis must have the catheter removed within 48 to 72 hours postinjury and a suprapubic cystostomy placed. If this is not accomplished, the ventral portion of the penis and urethra will slough, often resulting in a large soft tissue loss and a penile scrotal hypospadias.[20] This injury is repaired, as indicated in Figure 3.11, 6 to 8 months postinjury.

The most common long term complication of perineal burns is contracture formation. Contractures develop slowly and therefore a surgical

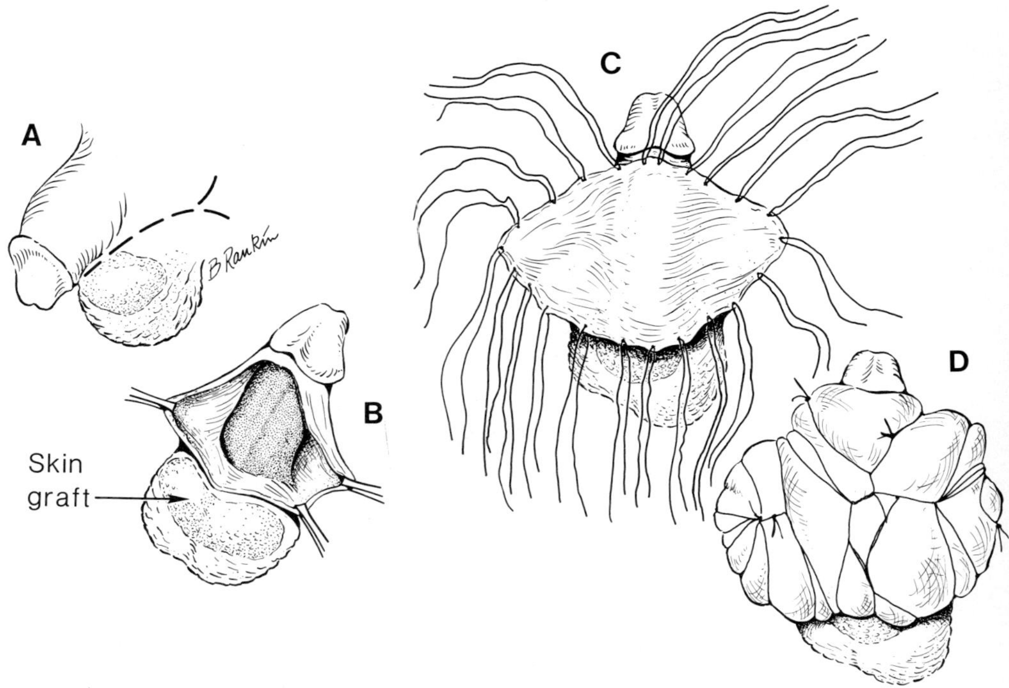

Figure 3.12. Release of genital contractures. *A*, the contracture has resulted in a short penile shaft which is immobile. A full thickness injury of the scrotum which required a split thickness skin graft in the immediate postburn period is illustrated. The incision to be made is outlined and is placed perpendicular to the line of contracture. It extends beneath the penis to the opposite side of the scrotum (not depicted). Darts are placed at either end of the incision. *B*, the defect created is extensive. The penis is released and assumes its normal length. *C*, thick split thickness skin is applied to the defect and sutured in place. *D*, the graft is stented by tying the sutures placed at the margin of the graft over cotton wadding.

EXTERNAL GENITALIA INJURIES

repair should not be performed for 8 to 12 months postburn at which time maturation of the scar is usually complete. The contracture is released by an incision placed perpendicular to the line of stress (Fig. 3.12). Darts are fashioned at each end of the incision to minimize development of margin contractures. A thick split thickness graft is obtained after the release, for often the size of the defect created is much larger than anticipated. The graft is sutured in place and stented for 5 to 7 days.

RADIATION INJURY

Radiation injury of the perineum is usually a complication of radiotherapy to the pelvis for malignant disease. The acute injury is manifested by erythema and edema. Chronic changes include atrophy of the skin, telangiectasias, hyperpigmentation, excoriation, and compromise of the small blood vessels in the skin and integument. The lesion is painful, itches, and occasionally progresses to frank ulceration. Conservative therapy is indicated initially; however, when skin loss and ulceration occur, it is rarely of any benefit. Split thickness grafts enjoy minimal success due to the poor vascularity of the underlying tissues. Defects created by radiation are best treated by excision and primary closure or by rotating uninjured tissue into the area to close the defect.[21,22] The latter may be accomplished with either myocutaneous or arterialized pedicle flaps.

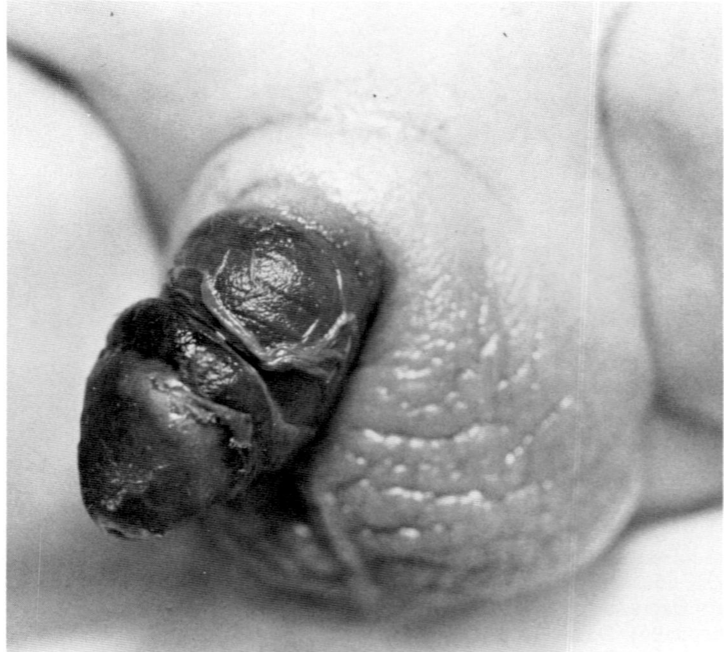

Figure 3.13. Penile skin slough in a newborn due to improper application of a Gomco clamp.

 TRAUMATIC INJURIES OF THE GENITOURINARY SYSTEM

CIRCUMCISION INJURIES

The injuries may involve the glans penis, the urethral meatus or the penile shaft (Fig. 3.13). Trauma to the glans is treated by primarily suturing the defect with fine reabsorbable suture. Small superficial skin losses will re-epithelialize spontaneously if the wound is kept uninfected. Large full thickness skin losses from the glans require the application of a split thickness skin graft. Meatal injuries may eventually result in scar formation with severe stenosis. A meatoplasty is then required. Excessive skin loss of the penile shaft is treated by the application of split thickness skin as described for avulsion injuries (Fig. 3.2).

REFERENCES

1. Balakrishnan, C. Scrotal avulsion: a new technique of reconstruction by split-skin graft. *Br. J. Plast. Surg. 9:*38, 1956.
2. Masters, F. W., and Robinson, D. W. The treatment of avulsions of the male genitalia. *J. Trauma 8:*430, 1968.
3. Schellhammer, P., and Donnelly, J. A mode of treatment for incarceration of the penis. *J. Trauma 13:*171, 1973.
4. Cohen, B. E., May, J. W., Jr., Daly, J. S. F., et al. Successful clinical replantation of an amputated penis by microneurovascular repair. *Plast. Reconstruct. Surg. 59:*276, 1977.
5. Tamai, S., Kakamura, Y., and Notomiya, Y. Microsurgical replantation of a completely amputated penis and scrotum. *Plast. Reconstruct. Surg. 60:*287, 1977.
6. Heymann, A. D., Bell-Thompson, J., Rathod, D. M., et al. Successful reimplantation of the penis using microvascular techniques. *J. Urol. 118:*879, 1977.
7. Engelman, E. R., Polito, G., Perley, J., et al. Traumatic amputation of the penis. *J. Urol. 112:*774, 1974.
8. McRoberts, W. J., Chapman, W. H., and Ansell, J. S. Primary anastomosis of the traumatically amputated penis: case report and summary of the literature. *J. Urol. 100:*751, 1968.
9. Taguchi, H., Saito, K., and Yamada, T. A simple method of total reconstruction of the penis. *Plast. Reconstruct. Surg. 60:*454, 1977.
10. Gilles, H., and Harrison, R. J. Congenital absence of the penis with embryological considerations. *Br. J. Plast. Surg. 1:*8, 1948.
11. Fleming, J. P. Reconstruction of the penis. *J. Urol 104:*213, 1970.
12. Evans, A. J. Buried skin-strip urethra in a tube pedicle phalloplasty. *Br. J. Plast. Surg. 16:*280, 1963.
13. Noe, J. M., Birdsell, D., and Laub, D. R. The surgical construction of male genitalia for the female-to-male transsexual. *Plast. Reconstruct. Surg. 53:*511, 1974.
14. Ovrum, E. Rupture of the penis. *Scand. J. Urol. Nephrol. 12:*83, 1978.
15. Hudson, M. J. K. Rupture of the corpus cavernosum of the penis. *Br. J. Clin. Pract. 29:*191, 1975.
16. Davies, D. M., and Mitchell, I. Fracture of the penis. *Br. J. Urol. 50:*426, 1978.
17. Gross, M., Arnold, T. L., and Waterhouse, K. Fracture of the penis: rationale of surgical management. *J. Urol. 106:*708, 1971.
18. Gross, M., Arnold, T. L., and Peters, P. Fracture of the penis with associated laceration of the urethra. *J. Urol. 117:*725, 1977.
19. Gross, M. Rupture of the testicle: the importance of early surgical treatment. *J. Urol. 101:*196, 1969.
20. McDougal, W. S., Peterson, H. D., Pruitt, B. A., et al. The thermally injured perineum. *J. Urol. 121:*320, 1979.
21. Barnes, W. E., Hoffman, G. W., and Pickrell, K. Surgical treatment of irradiation injuries of the perineum. *Surg. Gynecol. Obstet. 118:*1067, 1964.
22. Beare, R. L. B. Irradiation injuries of the perineum. *Br. J. Plast. Surg. 15:*22, 1962.

4

Urethral Injuries

The presentation, diagnosis, and therapy of urethral injuries are dependent upon the anatomic location of the injury and its extent. The urethral tear may result in a partial transection with maintenance of some mucosal continuity or a complete transection with separation of the two ends of the urethra. In the male, the location of the injury is classified as either an anterior urethral injury which includes the meatus, pendulous, and bulbous portions, or a posterior urethral injury in which case the prostato-membranous portion of the urethra is involved. Posterior urethral injuries are further subdivided according to where they occur in relation to the urogenital diaphragm. A urethral injury should be suspected when blood is seen at the meatus, if hematuria is present in the immediate postinjury voided specimen, or when the patient is unable to void. Urethral injuries should also be suspected in patients who have sustained pelvic fractures or straddle injuries.

The diagnosis is made by urethrography. Catheters should not be passed prior to urethrography in patients suspected of urethral injuries since partial disruptions may be inadvertently converted to complete disruptions. The technique of urethrography involves placing the patient in the right oblique position, 45° from the horizontal, with the right hip flexed and the left hip straight, inserting a 12 or 14 Foley catheter in the fossa navicularis, and instilling 10 cc of 10 to 20% radiocontrast. The injection is monitored under fluoroscopy and repeated as often as needed to make the proper diagnosis. In order to minimize periurethral tissue reaction and fibrosis, the amount of dye injected should be as little as is consistent with making an accurate diagnosis, and it should be water soluble and nonviscous. If fluoroscopy is unavailable, the roentgenogram should be taken during the injection so that a flow phase will be obtained. In partial ruptures, dye is found in the bladder and extravasated in the periurethral tissues adjacent to the injury site, whereas in complete ruptures, dye is found only in the periurethral tissues and not in the bladder[1] (Figs. 4.1 and 4.8).

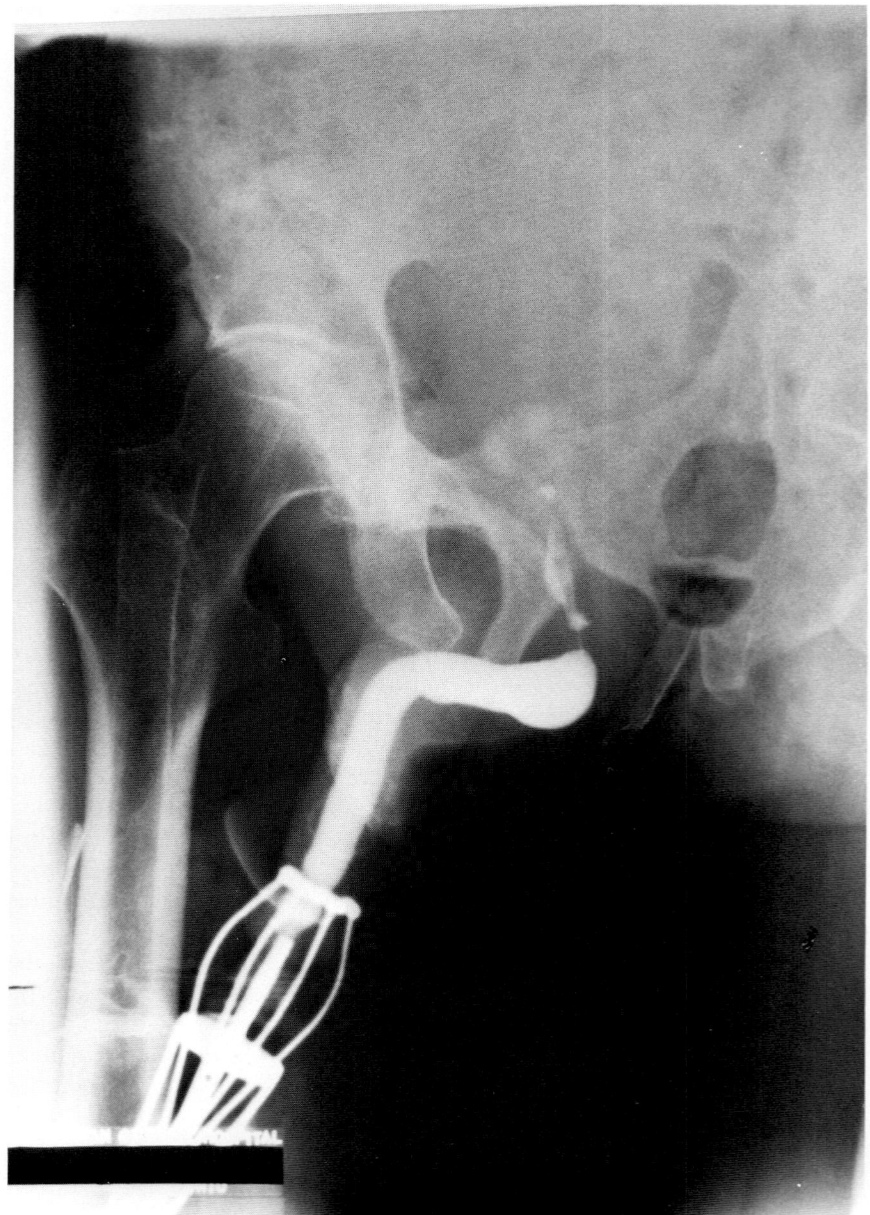

Figure 4.1. Urethrogram of a partial urethral tear. Notice that although there is extravasation of dye in the prostatomembranous portion of the urethra, some of it enters the bladder, confirming that the disruption is partial and not complete.

     TRAUMATIC INJURIES OF THE GENITOURINARY SYSTEM

ANTERIOR URETHRA

Etiology

The etiology of anterior urethral injuries includes blunt trauma, penetrating injury, urethral instrumentation, and indwelling catheters. Blunt-trauma such as straddle injuries or blows to the perineum may push the bulbous urethra against the pubic rami and cause a crush injury to this portion of the urethra. Injuries due to instrumentation—often as a consequence of transurethral resection—occur in the fixed portions of the urethra: meatus, at the level of the suspensory ligament and in the membranous portion. Catheters which remain indwelling block periurethral secretions and promote infection and scarring. They may result in pressure necrosis—often at the penile scrotal junction or in the pendulous urethra when a full thickness thermal injury to the ventrum of the shaft of the penis has been sustained. Chemicals used in the manufacture of catheters which have not been properly removed may serve as direct irritants to the urethra. This is more common in the smaller sized catheters since the chemical plasticizer which is used in the curing process may be difficult to completely remove from the small catheter.[2] The long term sequela of infections and chemical irritation is stricture formation. The stricture may cause further damage by resulting in spontaneous rupture proximally with periurethral extravasation (Fig. 4.2), abscess formation, necrosis, and rarely necrotizing gangrene.

Diagnosis

Anterior urethral injuries may present with blood at the meatus, a hematoma or tenderness on the shaft or at the base of the penis, hematuria, and inability to void. If Buck's fascia remains intact, the hematoma and extravasated urine will be confined to the shaft of the penis; however, if Buck's fascia is violated, blood and urine may follow the plane of Colles' fascia and involve the scrotum and anterior abdominal wall (Fig. 4.3). Urethrography makes the diagnosis and should be performed before a catheter is placed in the urethra.

Treatment

Partial disruptions may be successfully treated in two ways. A urethral catheter may be gently passed into the bladder, being careful not to traumatize the injured area. The area is drained if hematoma formation or extravasation is extensive using a penrose drain placed through a transverse incision in the penis which extends beneath Buck's fascia to the level of the urethra. The catheter is left indwelling for 2 to 3 weeks. Another method of treating partial disruptions of the anterior urethra is by the placement of a suprapubic cystostomy. The urethra is not manipulated; however, if extravasation or hematoma is extensive, the area is drained as described above. Using this latter modality of therapy, Pontes reported that 15 of 16 patients had an excellent result.[3]

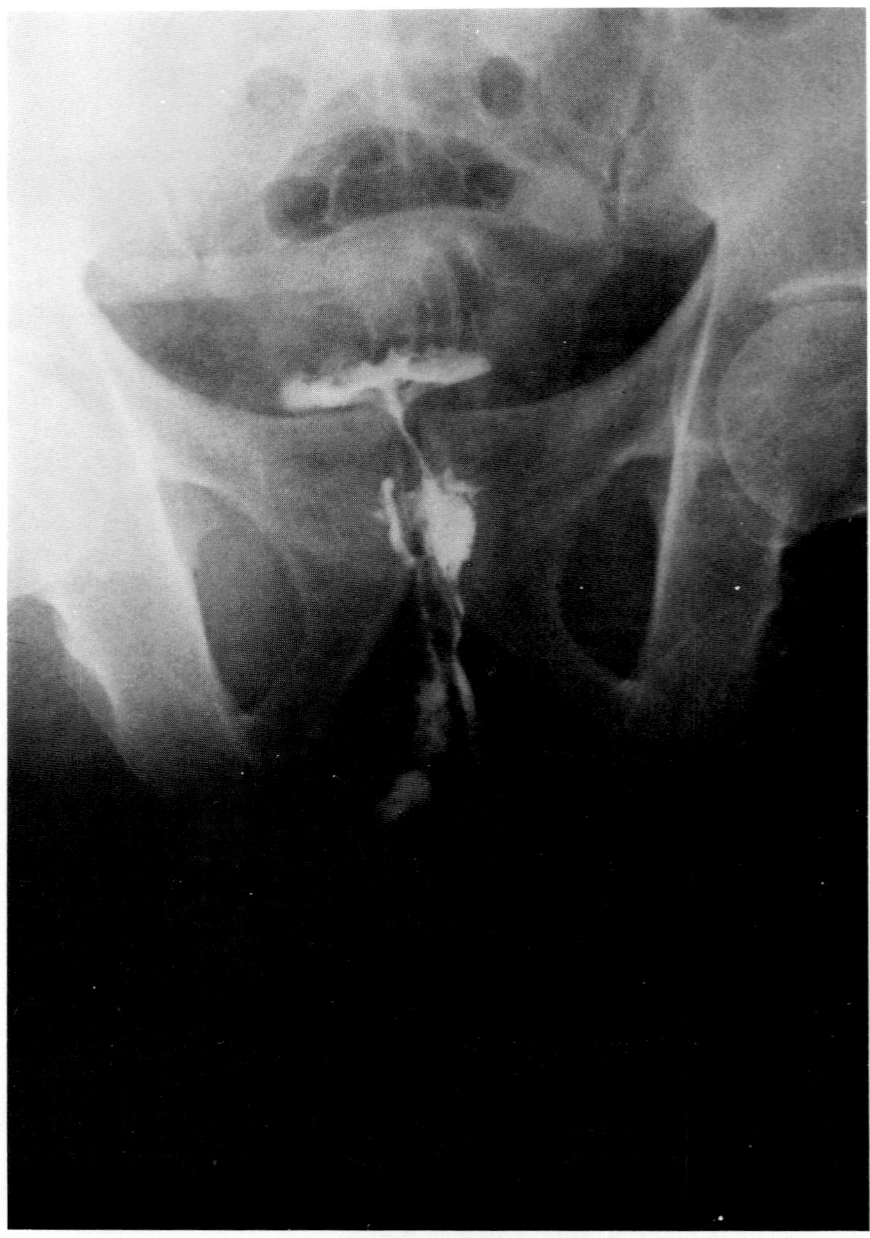

Figure 4.2. Urethrogram demonstrating a urethral rupture proximal to a urethral stricture with perineal extravasation.

Partial injuries of the anterior urethra which are small in extent, have little extravasation or hematoma formation, and in which Buck's fascia is intact are best treated with a urethral catheter. Larger injuries in which extravasation or hematoma formation is extensive and in which Buck's fascia is disrupted are appropriately managed either by suprapublic

     TRAUMATIC INJURIES OF THE GENITOURINARY SYSTEM

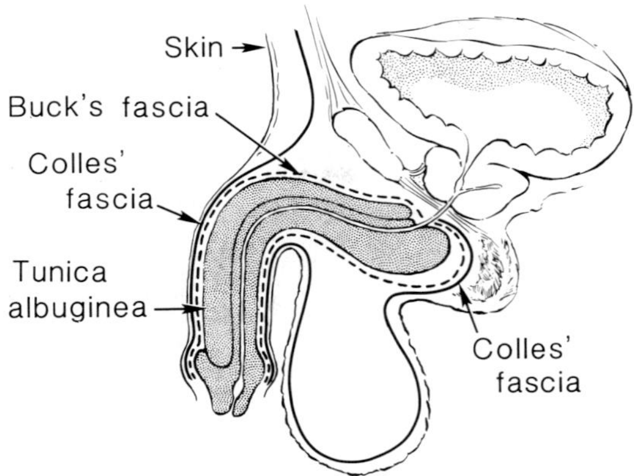

Figure 4.3. The fascial planes of the external genitalia are illustrated. Notice that if Buck's fascia remains intact, urethral extravasations are confined to the shaft of the penis; however, when this layer is disrupted, extravasated urine follows the plane of Colles' fascia and may enter the scrotum, perineum, and anterior abdominal wall.

diversion and local drainage or by transurethral catheter placement and local drainage.

Complete disruptions require a primary repair. A suprapubic cystostomy is placed. If the patient's condition does not warrant a prolonged surgical procedure, the urethral repair may be delayed until a more appropriate time; however, if the patient is stable, one should proceed with the repair. The urethra is mobilized by incising the fascia which adheres the corpus spongiosum to the corpus cavernosa. Bleeders are frequently found in this fascial attachment and should be ligated. The urethra is mobilized sufficiently so that after 1 to 2 cm are debrided, the ends may be anastomosed without tension on the suture line. Each end of the freshened urethra is spatulated (the spatulation on one end is made 180° from that on the other) and sewn together with interrupted 4-0 chromic. This results in an oblique suture line which reduces the chances of a symptomatic stricture developing from a circumferential scar (Fig. 4.4). The anastomosis is drained and may be stented or left unstented. Both methods result in a satisfactory outcome. However, if a stent is preferred it should be of modest caliber so as not to put pressure on the anastomosis. A fenestrated catheter in which multiple holes are cut in the shaft of the catheter has been proposed by Turner-Warwick[4] (Fig. 4.5). This catheter allows for drainage of the periurethral secretions and is said to result in less periurethral inflammation and infection. The urethral catheter should be sewn to the glans penis, secured to the suprapubic tube by means of a suture, or its security in the bladder assured by means of a suture placed through the urethral catheter tip and brought out on the abdomen adjacent to the suprapubic tube. This will minimize the chances of inadvertent dislodgement and with the latter two methods—should dislodgement occur, the urethral catheter may be replaced with minimal trauma.

URETHRAL INJURIES

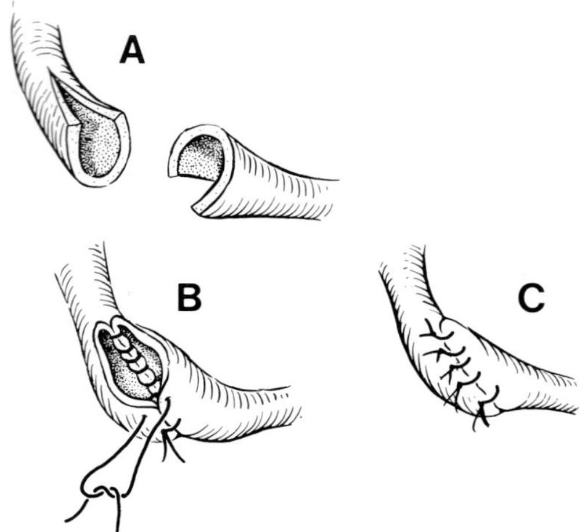

Figure 4.4. Repair of traumatic injuries of the urethra requires adequate debridement of all devitalized tissue. The two ends of the disrupted urethra are freed and spatulated, one on the opposite side from the other, *A*. The anastomosis is performed with fine interrupted resorbable suture resulting in a tension free oblique suture line, *B* and *C*.

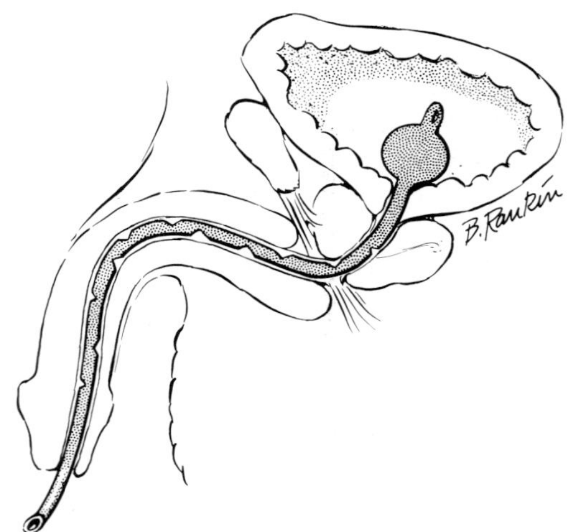

Figure 4.5. A fenestrated catheter drains the periurethral secretions thereby reducing the chance of periurethral inflammation and stricture formation.

Complications

Complications of anterior urethral injuries include strictures, fistulae, necrotizing infection, and abscess formation. Strictures and fistula formation can be minimized by atraumatic passage of catheters, by mobilizing sufficient urethra so that the urethral anastomosis can be performed without tension on the suture line, and by preventing infection through proper drainage and appropriate use of antibiotics. Periurethral extravasations can result in abscess formation and, on rare occasions, a necrotiz-

 TRAUMATIC INJURIES OF THE GENITOURINARY SYSTEM

ing soft tissue gangrene which is rapidly progressive and often times fatal (Fournier's Gangrene, Fig. 4.6). Microaerophilic streptococcus and *Staphylococcus aureus* are classically the responsible organisms. The process is very aggressive and begins as a localized discoloration on the perineum which, over a period of several hours, rapidly progresses to involve the penile, scrotal and, finally, the abdominal wall skin in the gangrenous process. The patient becomes toxic and his cardiovascular system becomes unstable. The disease entity is a surgical emergency for even under the best of circumstances mortality is exceedingly high. The blood pressure must be supported and broad spectrum antibiotics need to be given intravenously. The patient is taken directly to the operating room where a radical debridement is performed. Often large cutaneous defects are created and the penis and testes are denuded. Due to their separate blood

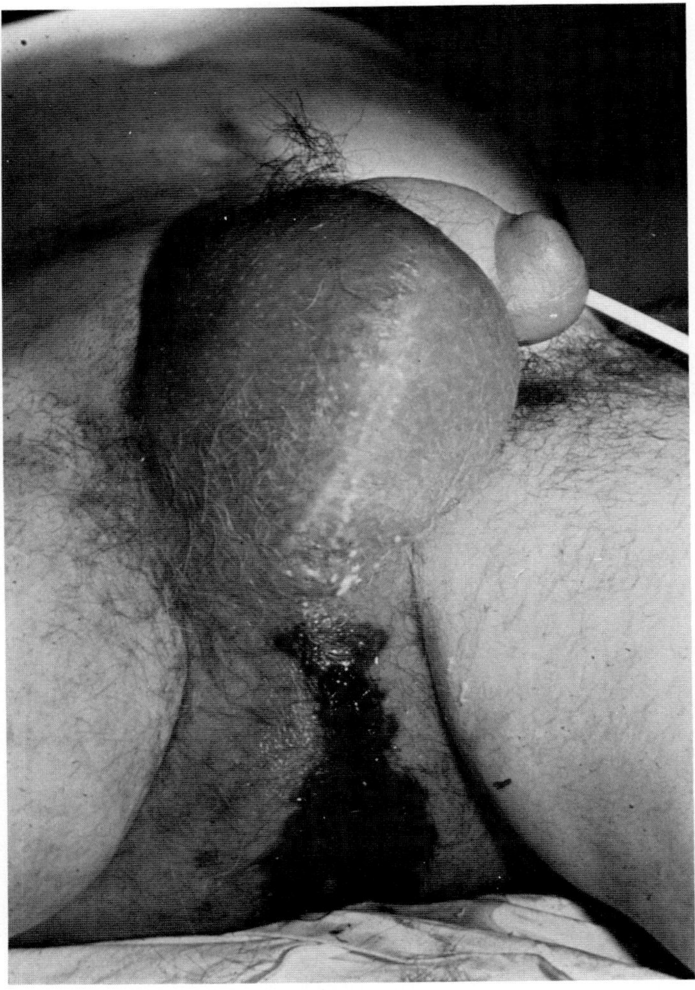

Figure 4.6.   Necrotizing gangrene of the perineum (Fournier's Gangrene) occurring as a consequence of a ruptured urethra.

supply, the deep tissues of these structures are invariable viable (Fig. 4.7). The wound should be left open and packed. The patient is returned to the operating room, anesthetized, and debrided on a daily basis until no more necrotic tissue can be found on two consecutive days. At this point, the testes are implanted in the thighs and the defect covered with autograph or homograph followed by autograph. Reconstruction of the scrotum may be performed at a later date as described in Chapter 3.

POSTERIOR URETHRA

Etiology

Posterior urethral injuries usually occur as a result of automobile accidents or crush injuries and rarely as a result of penetrating trauma. They are often associated with pelvic fractures. Indeed, 90% of these injuries have concomitant pelvic fractures. Conversely, 10% of pelvic fractures are associated with posterior urethral injuries. Unfortunately, impotence is not an uncommon sequelae. Twenty to 40% of patients with severe pelvic fractures and posterior urethral disruptions will be impotent (the more comminuted the pelvic fracture, the greater the chance of impotence).[5, 6]

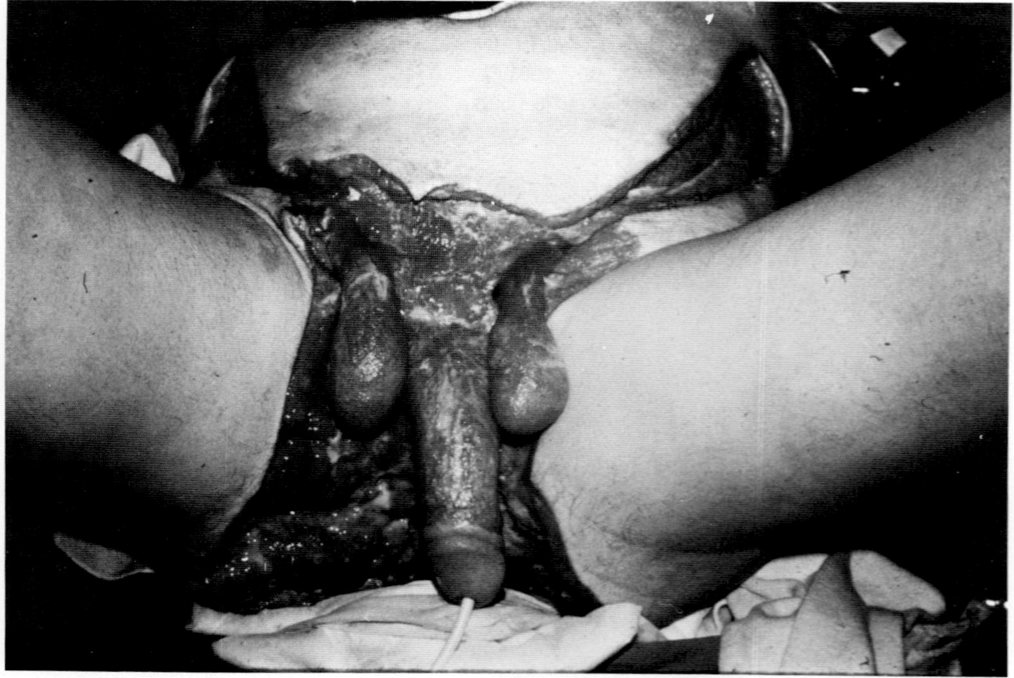

Figure 4.7. Extensive debridement is required in managing patients with necrotizing gangrene of the perineum. Notice that the testicles are denuded but remain viable due to their separate blood supply from that of the perineal skin.

 TRAUMATIC INJURIES OF THE GENITOURINARY SYSTEM

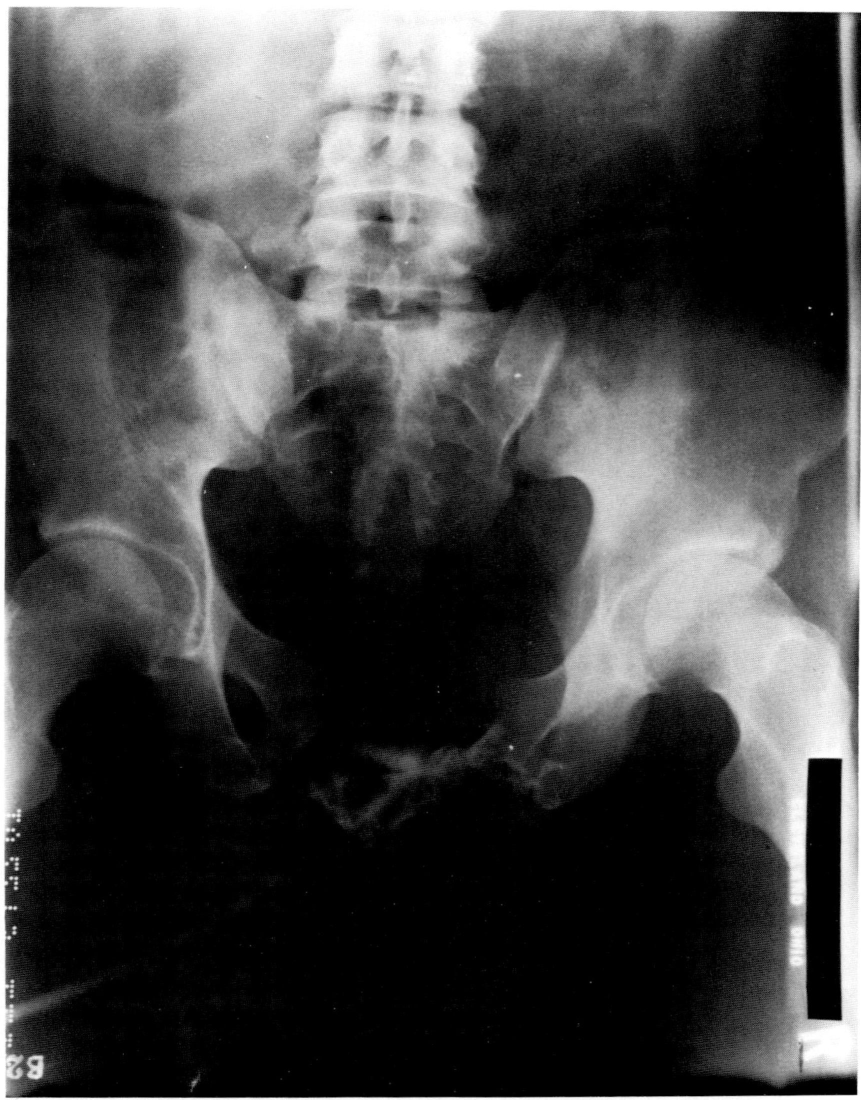

Figure 4.8. Urethrogram of a complete disruption of the posterior urethra. Notice that dye does not enter the bladder confirming the complete nature of the urethral disruption. Note the diastasis of the symphasis pubis.

Diagnosis

This injury should be suspected when the patient has sustained a pelvic fracture and there is blood at the meatus, the patient is unable to void, the prostate is displaced cephalad, there is a perineal hematoma or the bladder appears as a cephalad displaced inverted tear drop structure on intravenous pyelography. On occasion, cephalad displacement of the prostate and an inverted tear drop appearance of the bladder may occur in the presence of extensive hematoma formation without a concomitant ure-

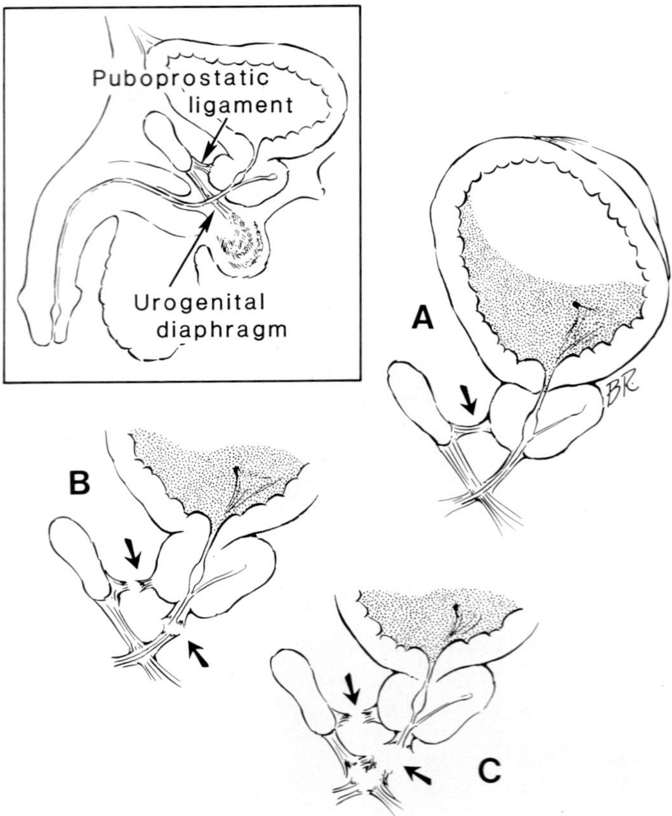

Figure 4.9.   Classification of posterior urethral injuries according to their location with respect to the urogenital diaphragm. *A*, the prostatomembranous urethra is stretched but remains intact. *B*, the prostatomembranous urethra is disrupted above the urogenital diaphragm. The puboprostatic ligament is also disrupted. *C*, the prostatomembranous urethra is disrupted both above and below the urogenital diaphragm. The puboprostatic ligament is disrupted. *D*, a urethogram of a prostatomembranous urethral disruption of Type III. Notice that the extravasated dye is above and below the urogenital diaphragm.

thral injury. The urethrogram is diagnostic and must be performed before any attempt is made at passing a catheter (Fig. 4.8). These injuries are subclassified into one of three groups depending upon the findings of the urethrogram[7] (Fig. 4.9). Type I: The prostate or urogenital diaphragm is dislocated but the membranous urethra is merely stretched and not severed. There is no extravasation of dye. The treatment involves urethral catheter placement for 10 to 14 days. Type II: The membranous urethra is ruptured above the urogenital diaphragm at the apex of the prostate. The urethrogram shows an intact bulbous urethra, intrapelvic extravasation, and no perineal extravasation. Type III: The membranous urethra is ruptured above and below the urogenital diaphragm. This is the most common type of disruption. The urethrogram reveals extravasation into

     TRAUMATIC INJURIES OF THE GENITOURINARY SYSTEM

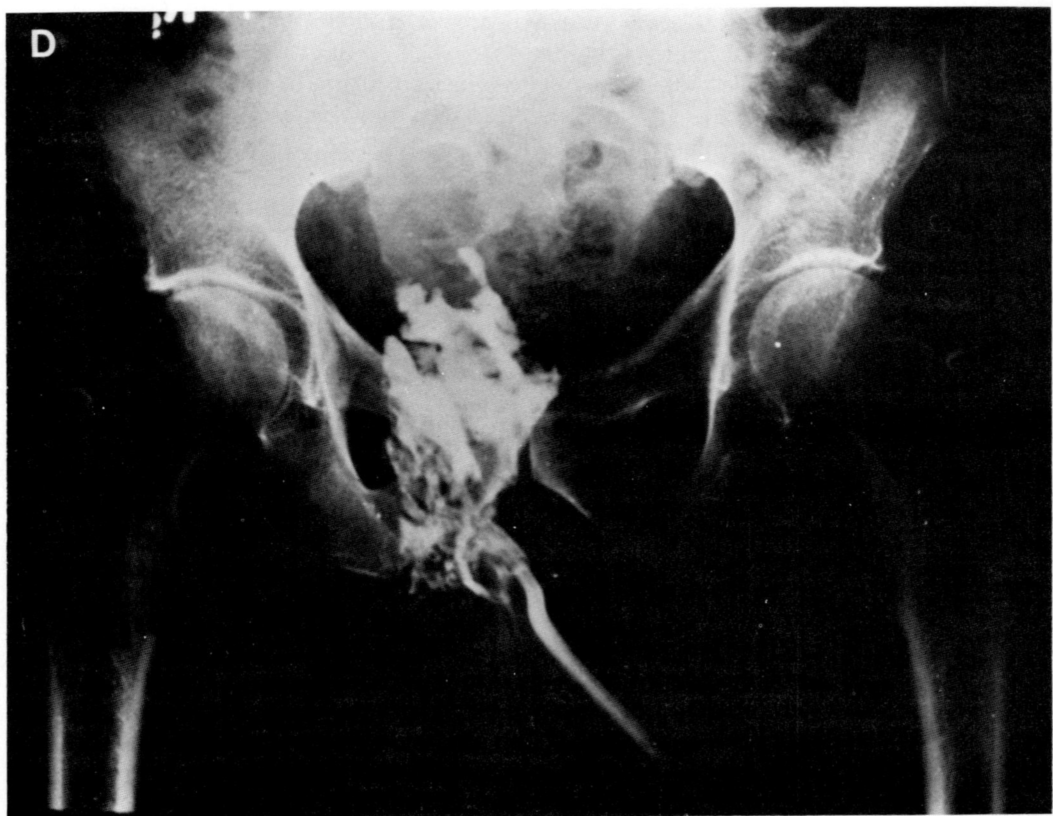

Figure 4.9*D*

the perineum only. No contrast is seen above the urogenital diaphragm. These disruptions may be partial or complete. When the disruption is complete, the puboprostatic ligaments are usually lacerated and the bladder neck is in spasm so that very little urinary extravasation occurs. Hematoma formation is usually considerable. The bleeding ceases when enough pressure has been created by the expanding hematoma to tamponade the vessels. Indeed, suprapubic exploration in the presence of a severely fractured pelvis often results in brisk bleeding which is difficult to control.

Partial disruptions are treated by a suprapubic cystotomy, urethral catheter placement, and drainage. Both catheters are tied to each other to prevent inadvertent urethral catheter dislodgement. The urethral catheter should be left in place for 2 to 4 weeks. If left indwelling for shorter periods, there is a high incidence of subsequent stricture formation. Partial disruptions of the prostatic urethra, often a consequence of penetrating injuries or transurethral manipulations, may be repaired primarily if they can be approached without the need for extensive dissections. A suprapubic cystostomy and transurethral catheter are placed as described above. Immediate repair of these injuries markedly reduces postinjury drainage, periurethral and perivesical fibrosis, and morbidity.

URETHRAL INJURIES   69

Complete disruptions may be treated in two ways: by immediate repair and by delayed repair. Immediate repair requires that the patient is stable and that few other traumatic injuries coexist. In severely comminuted pelvic fractures, this approach may result in excessive blood loss and poor visibility during the procedure. Consequently, patients amenable to immediate repair are those who are stable and do not have extensive associated injuries, a severely comminuted pelvis, or pre-existing urethral disease. The bladder is opened, the hematoma is evacuated and loose bone is removed. Both ends of the severed urethra are located either with interlocking sounds (Fig. 4.10) or by catheters passed proximally and distally. The prostate and bladder neck must not be mobilized for, if this is done, the patient will almost assuredly be impotent. A catheter is placed from the meatus into the bladder, thereby re-establishing urethral continuity. No attempt is made to reapproximate the severed urethra with sutures, for they will tear out and the dissection required will increase the potential for impotence. The prostate may be pulled onto the urogenital diaphragm, thereby reapproximating the severed urethra by means of traction sutures placed through either side of the prostate, brought out the perineum and tied over bumpers.[9] The urethral catheter is fenestrated and tied to the suprapubic catheter (Fig. 4.11). Of seven patients treated

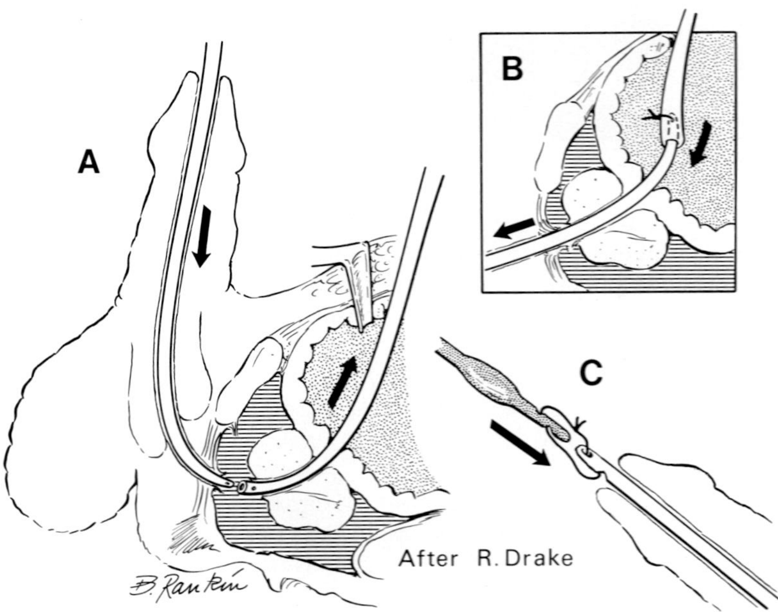

Figure 4.10. Interlocking sounds may be used to locate the two ends of a severed urethra and restore continuity. *A*, the sounds are placed into the urethra, one through the meatus and the other through the bladder neck and brought together. *B*, the urethral sound is guided into the bladder and a catheter sutured to its end. The catheter is drawn from the bladder out the meatus. *C*, a Foley catheter is attached to the bladder catheter and the Foley drawn into the bladder.

 TRAUMATIC INJURIES OF THE GENITOURINARY SYSTEM

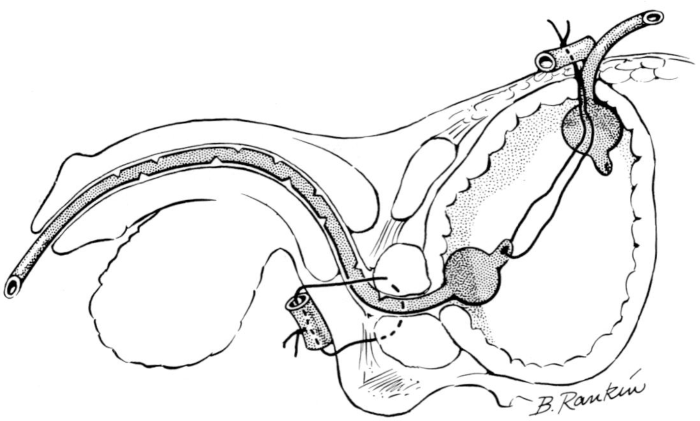

Figure 4.11. In complete disruptions of the prostatomembranous urethra, the prostate may be returned to its normal position and secured in place by passing sutures through it and then out the perineum. The sutures are tied over rubber bumpers on the perineum and urethral continuity maintained with a fenestrated Foley catheter. Notice that the urethral catheter has been secured by a suture placed through it and brought out on the abdomen over a rubber bumper.

by this method, all had excellent results and all were asymptomatic; two have been followed for more than 5 years.[10] Alternatively, the severed urethra may be reapproximated by applying traction to the urethral catheter, providing the urogenital diaphragm is intact to provide support.[11] The catheter is held at 45° by the weight of 200 to 500 g for 4 to 6 days (Fig. 4.12). The angle realigns the ends in their normal anatomic position and the specified weight prevents pressure necrosis on the bladder neck. Too much weight will cause necrosis of the bladder neck, loss of the internal sphincter, and loss of continence since it is the internal sphincter which provides for continence in patients with posterior urethral disruptions. Twenty of 22 patients treated by this method have had satisfactory results over the long term.[11] The advantages of immediate repair over delayed repair include a reduced morbidity and a reduced incidence of stricture over the short term. A disadvantage, however, is that when a long term stricture does develop, it is generally more difficult to repair (Fig. 4.13). The incidence of incontinence from several series is about 15%, the incidence of impotence is about 33%, and the incidence of long term stricture formation is about 32%.[5, 6, 12] These statistics may be biased, however, since it is unclear whether extensive mobilization of the prostate and bladder neck were performed. When dissection about the prostate and bladder neck is kept to a minimum, the incidence of incontinence, impotence, and stricture formation are reduced.

Delayed repair involves initially placing a suprapubic cystostomy and avoiding any manipulation of the urethra. Since 100% of the complete disruptions develop a stricture, the definitive urethral repair is performed 3 to 6 months later. As the hematoma resorbs, the prostate returns to its normal position; however, occasionally it remains distracted, making the subsequent repair exceedingly difficult. The advantages of this approach

URETHRAL INJURIES   71

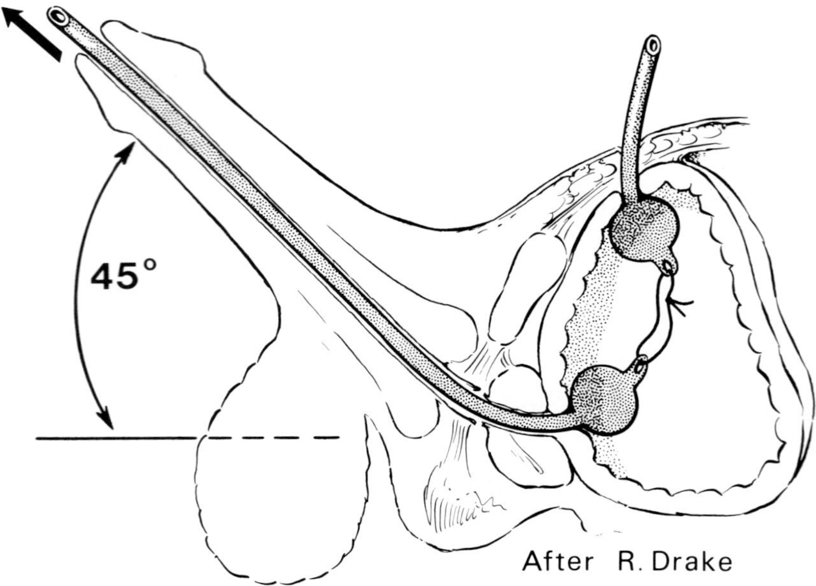

Figure 4.12. Complete prostatomembranous urethral disruptions may also be realigned and held in place by placing traction on the urethral catheter. The catheter is maintained at a 45° angle thereby restoring the normal anatomy. This procedure is not applicable when the urogenital diaphragm is markedly disrupted for if it does not provide support, the prostate will be pulled too far caudally.

include less chance of infecting the hematoma, thereby resulting in extensive periurethral fibrosis, a low incidence of impotence (about 7%), avoidance of converting a partial disruption into a complete one, and a low incidence of incontinence. These statistics, however, exclude those patients who are impotent by virtue of their original injury, and, therefore, it is difficult to compare the incidence of complications arising from delayed repair to those occurring subsequent to a direct primary repair. The disadvantages include a 100% incidence of stricture formation requiring repair, the prolonged morbidity of a suprapubic catheter, and an incidence of recurrent stricture requiring surgical repair of 13%.[12] The delayed repair is the procedure of choice in patients who have a severely comminuted pelvis, multiple associated injuries, or a prior history of urethral disease.

It is our practice in managing complete prostatomembranous disruptions to realign the severed ends over a urethral catheter and perform a suprapubic cystostomy in the immediate postinjury period. The catheters are tied together to prevent inadvertent dislodgement. Care is taken not to explore or dissect the retropubic area nor to place any traction on the urethral catheter. The urethral catheter is left indwelling for 4 to 6 weeks. With this approach, we have two patients who void satisfactorily through the penis and have required no subsequent operative procedures. Those who develop a stricture are repaired transpubically at 6 to 8 months postinjury. It is our impression that the repair is facilitated in those in

     TRAUMATIC INJURIES OF THE GENITOURINARY SYSTEM

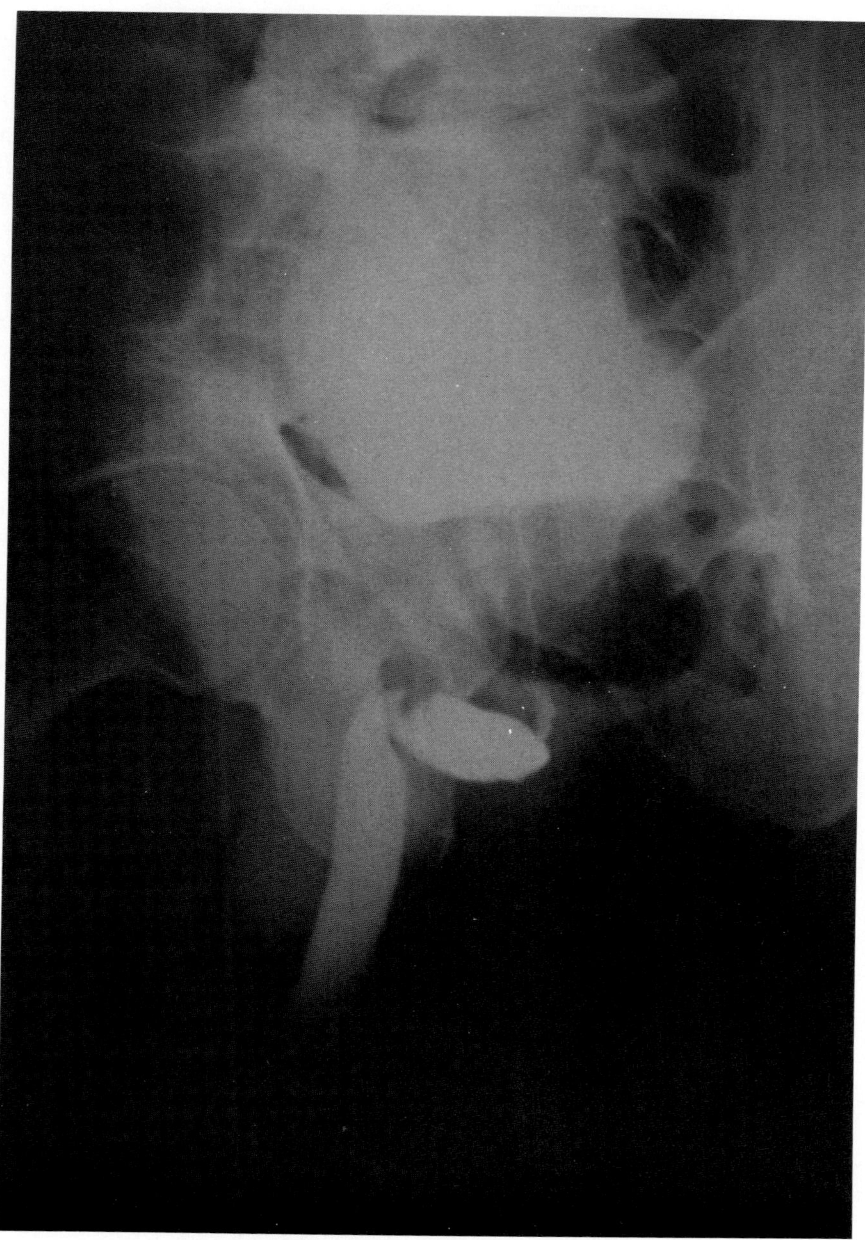

Figure 4.13. Urethrogram 6 months postinjury in a patient who sustained a prostatomembranous urethral disruption treated initially by a suprapubic cystostomy and urethral catheter placement. The bladder remained distracted from the urethra and a long neourethral stricture developed.

whom the urethra has been realigned immediately postinjury and the incidence of complications comparable to those managed by suprapubic cystostomy alone.

Transpubic Section and Symphysiotomy

In the delayed repair, the stricture is first approached through the perineum. This approach is satisfactory for most cases; however, if proper exposure cannot be obtained, which is usually the case in supradiaphragmatic injuries or injuries where the severed ends are separated by a wide gap, a combined anterior and perineal approach is used. Prior to surgery, the stricture is evaluated by simultaneous urethrography and cystography since the position and length of the stricture must be known preoperatively. The patient is placed in the St. Mark's position. The distal urethra is approached through the perineum and freed for a considerable length (Waterhouse advocates freeing the urethra to the glans penis[13]). Attention is turned to the suprapubic area where a lower abdominal midline incision is made extending over the symphysis to the root of the penis (Fig. 4.14). The incision provides exposure for either a transpubic section or symphysiotomy. The symphysis is identified and, using a subperiosteal dissection, the attachments of the pyramidalis and recti are cleaned from the pubis. The retropubic space is entered. The periosteum is stripped from the caudal aspect of the symphysis. The suspensory ligament of the penis is divided and the dorsal vein of the penis is identified. This may also require ligation and division. The symphysis is encircled by developing a subperiosteal plane on its inferior aspect. This prevents injury to the venous plexus in the space of Retzius. By staying adjacent to bone (beneath the periosteum) the urogenital diaphragm is pushed posteriorly opening a space beneath the pubis. A Gigli saw is passed on either side and a trapezoidal piece of bone is removed (an osteotome may be used in place of the Gigli saw). If a symphysiotomy is desired, a single midline cut with the Gigli saw is made and a self retaining retractor is placed between the severed pubis. As the pubis is forcibly separated, the anterior and superior sacroiliac ligaments may be torn.[14] On occasion, their rupture may result in prolonged postoperative back pain. Exuberant new bone formation about the injured area may obscure the urethra and should be removed. The proximal urethra is mobilized and an oblique end to end repair may be performed or the distal urethra may be telescoped into the prostatic urethra and sutured in place (Badendock). The latter procedure results in infertility since the ejaculatory ducts are obstructed by the telescoped urethra. The periosteum is closed. The resected bone results in a dead space which may either be left empty or filled with a rectus muscle flap or an omental pedicle flap. Prolonged drainage from the dead space occurs on occasion and is more common if the space has not been filled with omentum or rectus muscle. Postoperatively, the patient should remain in bed for 5 days. There is no pelvic instability with this approach and no loss of potency. In several series, no patient was rendered impotent by the procedure. Some patients experience pain in the lower extremities postoperatively, but this quickly passes.

 TRAUMATIC INJURIES OF THE GENITOURINARY SYSTEM

Pedicle Flaps

Wound drainage, infection, periurethral fibrosis, and recurrent stricture formation can be minimized in patients undergoing a delayed repair of a posterior urethral disruption by filling the periurethral dead space with a pedicle flap. If a rectus muscle flap is employed, care must be exercised to preserve the inferior epigastric vessels during mobilization of the rectus muscle. The omental pedicle is an excellent tissue to place about anastomoses and in cavities to fill dead space since it does well in infected, irradiated, and poorly vascularized areas, maintains pliability, and aids in resolving infection and preventing fibrosis. The construction of an omental pedicle graft requires a knowledge of its vascular supply (Fig. 4.15). The omentum derives its blood supply from the right and left gastroepiploic arteries which course immediately beneath the greater curve of the stomach and anastomose with each other in the midline. Three major vessels arise from the gastroepiploic and course caudally to form an anastomotic arcade at the distal end: the right, middle, and left omental vessels. The right and left omental vessels arise at the lateral boarder of the omental apron, whereas the middle omental vessel arises in the midline. On occasion, an accessory omental vessel may arise lateral to the right omental artery. The omental flap is created by severing the omental attachment to the transverse colon along its avascular plane. The omentum is freed from the stomach being careful to preserve the gastroepiploic arch and include it within the omental apron. The short gastric vessels are individually ligated on the stomach side with fine silk and on the omental side with reabsorbable suture. Individual vessel ligation is important for mass ligatures will result in foreshortening of the pedicle. Resorbable suture must be employed on that portion of the omentum which will come in contact with the urinary tract since infection and crystal precipitation will be encouraged and perpetuated should nonreabsorbable material be employed. Care must be taken not to tear any of the vessels for large hematoma formation in the omentum will occur and obscure the dissection and jeopardize the flap. The left gastroepiploic is transected at the lateral margin thereby basing the vascular supply on the right gastroepiploic since this vessel is often slightly larger than the left. If necessary, however, the flap may be based on the left gastroepiploic. The hepatocolic ligament is transected and the right colon mobilized medially. The omental flap is retroperitonealized by rotating the flap caudally and placing it beneath the mesentary of the right colon. The colon is replaced in its normal anatomic position. Generally sufficient length will be obtained by the single section of the left gastroepiploic. However, occasionally, additional length is required in which case an incision is made through the gastroepiploic vessel extending caudally to the inferior vascular arch between the right and middle omental vessels. Care must be taken to preserve the distal arch which connects the right omental vessel to the middle and left omental vessels if viability of the distal apron is to be maintained. This maneuver will provide more than enough length for pelvic and urethral use.

URETHRAL INJURIES

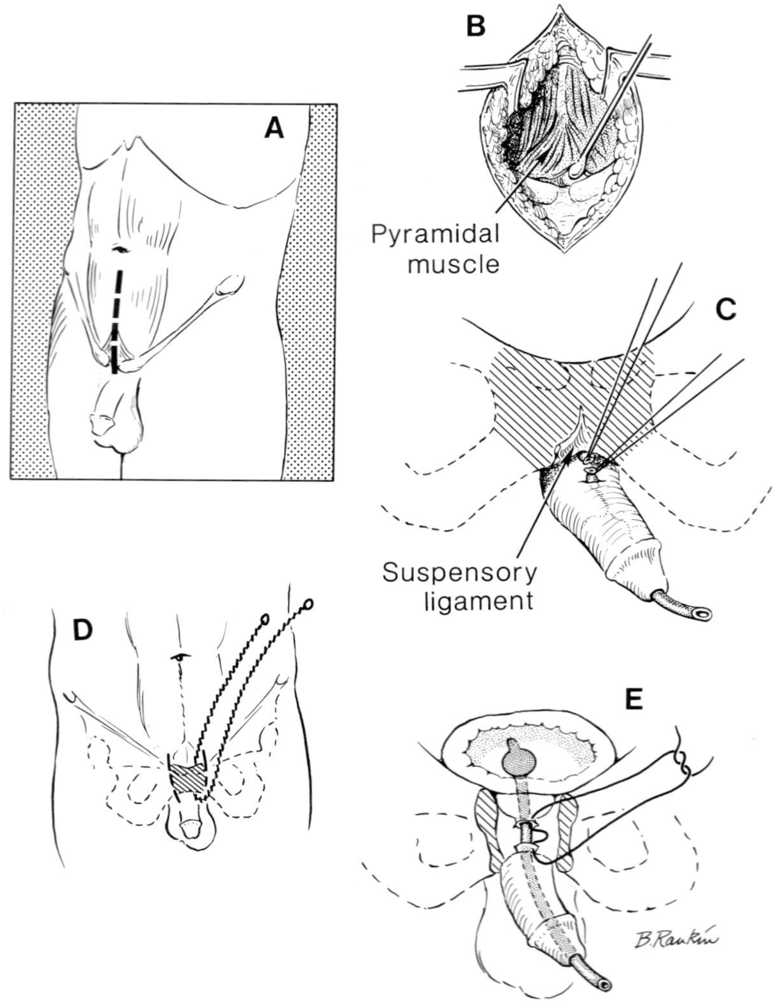

Figure 4.14. Transpubic approach for repair of the posterior urethra. *A*, the incision extends to the base of the penis. *B*, the insertions of the pyramidalis and rectus are cleared from the symphasis by a subperiosteal dissection. *C*, the suspensory ligament of the penis and the superficial dorsal vein are severed and the periosteum cleared from beneath the symphasis. The urogenital diaphragm is pushed caudad with the periosteum. *D*, using a Gigli saw, the bone is resected, *E*, the urethral anastomosis may be performed with ease. *F*, voiding cystourethrogram of a patient who had a prostatomembranous urethral disruption repaired 6 months following the accident by the transpubic approach.

Complications

The complications of posterior urethral disruptions include stricture formation, incontinence, and impotence. Although the delayed repair appears to result in a lesser incidence of these complications from reported series in the literature, the series are not comparable nor prospective. In our experience, when the immediate repair is reserved for the stable

TRAUMATIC INJURIES OF THE GENITOURINARY SYSTEM

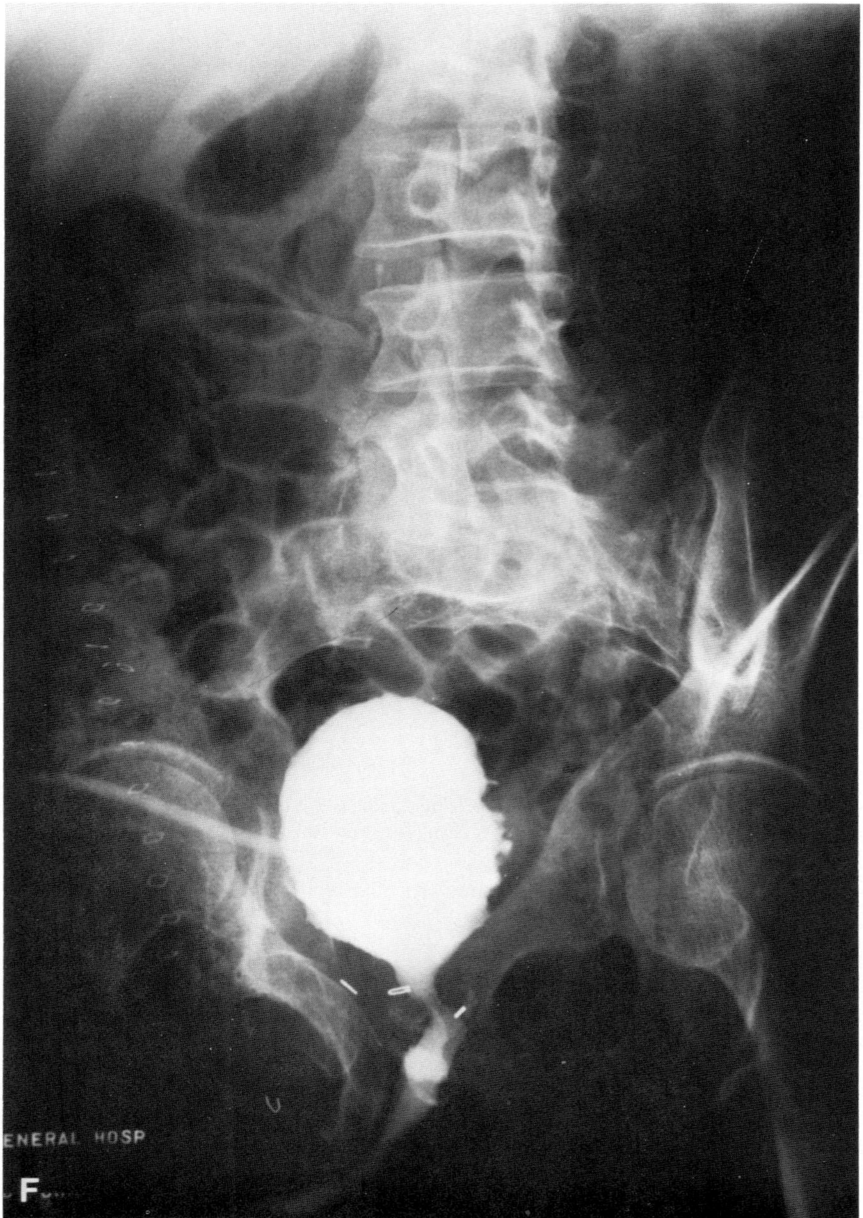

Figure 4.14F.

patient who does not have extensive associated injuries, a prior history of urethral disease or a severely comminuted pelvis, the incidence of these complications is about the same, provided dissection about the bladder neck and prostate are avoided.

It should be noted that continence in these patients is dependent upon the internal sphincter and that anything which will interfer with its action will likely produce incontinence. Thus, patients who require a prostatec-

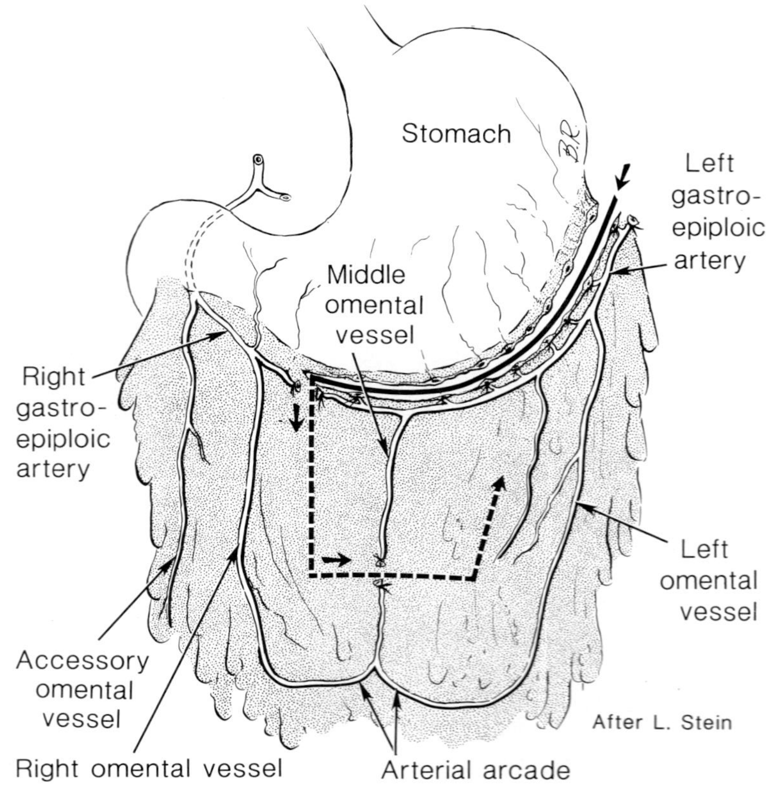

Figure 4.15. Omental pedicle flap. The vasculature is depicted and the *solid* and *dotted lines* illustrate the proper incision for creation of the vascularized pedicle.

tomy later in life must be warned about the likelihood of postpostratectomy incontinence.

RUPTURE OF THE FEMALE URETHRA

Rupture of the female urethra is an exceedingly rare injury. Perhaps this is because it is more mobile than the male urethra.[15] The prepubertal female is more prone to this injury than is the adult. It is most often a consequence of an automobile accident, however, rarely it may be due to penetrating trauma. The vagina is usually injured as well, perhaps explaining why a urethral vaginal fistula develops in almost all cases. As healing occurs, urethral stenosis commonly develops. If the urethral vaginal fistula is proximal to the sphincter the patient is incontinent.

Treatment

If possible, these injuries should be repaired immediately. The hematoma is evacuated, the bladder returned to its normal position, and urethral continuity re-established with a catheter. The catheter is tied to the suprapubic tube and may be placed on gentle traction if necessary to

     TRAUMATIC INJURIES OF THE GENITOURINARY SYSTEM

keep the distracted ends approximated. The vaginal lacerations should also be primarily repaired. Placement of a suprapubic tube as the sole form of treatment is acceptable if instability of the patient or other associated injuries make manipulation of the pelvic injury inadvisable or as a temporizing procedure until the experienced urologist can provide definitive care.

Complications

Complications include stricture, fistulae, and incontinence. If a low urethral vaginal fistula develops with no obstruction and the patient is continent, no further therapy is indicated as these are most difficult to correct and are often met with failure.[16] If the fistula is proximal, it is dissected free, the vaginal mucosa separated, and the urethra repaired. A bulbocavernosus flap, or omental pedicle, or a labial pedicle flap may be used to interpose tissue between vagina and urethra (Fig. 4.16). With the former two, the vaginal epithelium is closed over the interposed tissue. Bladder neck contractures also commonly develop and are treated by the standard Y-V plasty technique.

SLOUGH OF THE FEMALE URETHRA

Etiology

Slough of part of the female urethra may be due to obstetric trauma, automobile accidents, irradiation, gynecologic surgery, failed urethral diverticular repair, lymphopathiavenereum, and vulvourethral malignancies. The patient's continence is dependent upon the location of the slough in relation to the sphincter.

Treatment

The repair involves raising vaginal flaps and circumscribing the fistula. The fistula is closed with fine reabsorbable suture over a urethral catheter. Soft tissue is placed over the repair beneath the vaginal mucosa by utilizing either a Martinis flap (bulbocavernosus muscle)[17] or an omental pedicle graft, and the vaginal skin is closed. If the vaginal wall is scared or the tissue is of poor quality, a labial skin flap should be rotated to cover the repaired urethra (Fig. 4.16). If incontinence is a problem, an anterior suspension is performed at a later date. In 50 patients with urethral slough treated by this technique, 74% were cured, 14% were improved, and 12% remained unchanged.[18]

URETHRAL INJURIES IN CHILDHOOD

Anterior Urethra

The anterior urethra in children is rarely injured. On those occasions when the pendulous urethra is injured, it is usually a consequence of penetrating trauma, whereas injuries of the bulbous urethra often result

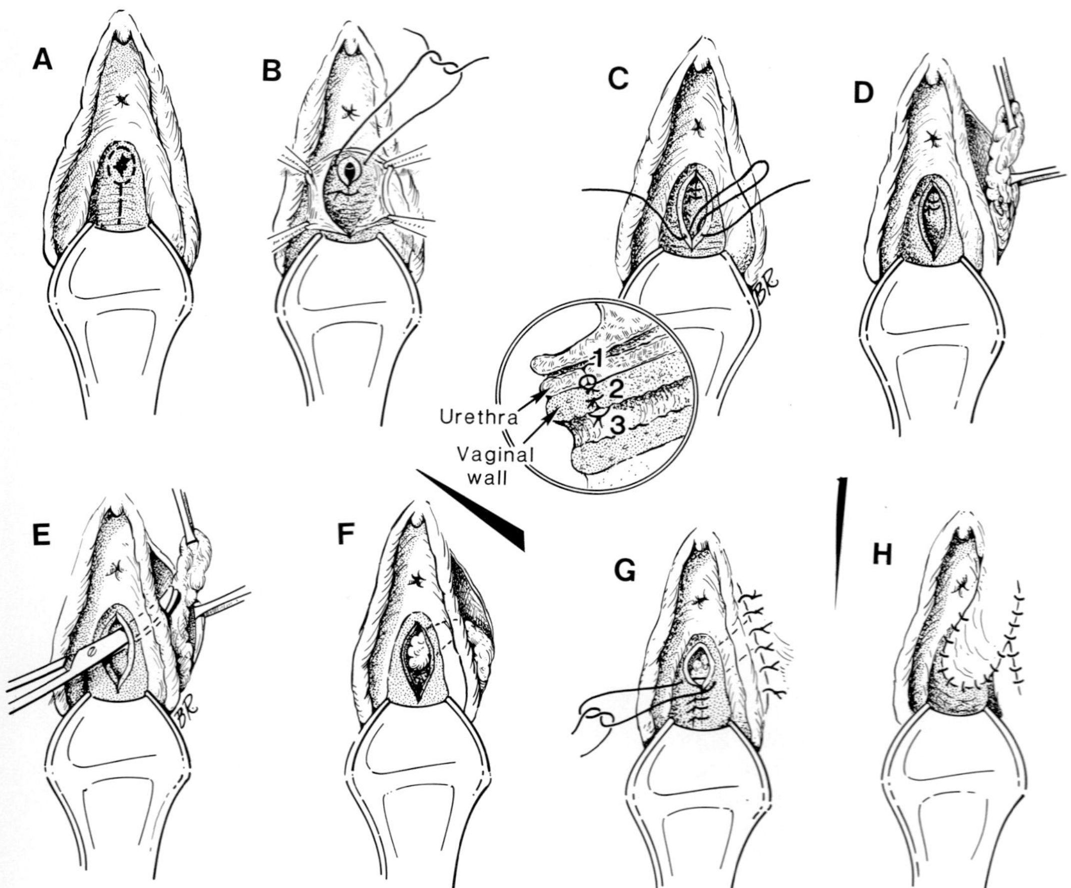

Figure 4.16. Repair of urethral injuries in females. *A*, urethral vaginal fistula to be circumscribed and excised is illustrated. The incision is depicted by the *dotted lines*. *B*, vaginal mucosal flaps are elevated. The urethral fistula margins have been excised and the urethral wall repaired with interrupted 5-0 chromic suture. *C*, the vaginal mucosa and subcutaneous tissue are closed in layers over the repaired urethra. Insert depicts lateral view of repair. *D*, healthy tissue may be interposed between the urethra and vaginal mucosa to insure a greater chance of a successful repair. A bulbocavernosus flap is mobilized by incising the labia majora. *E*, a subcutaneous tunnel is formed from the site of the urethral repair to the mobilized bulbocavernosus. *F*, the bulbocavernosus tissue is interposed over the urethral repair. *G*, the vaginal mucosa is closed thereby resulting in separation of the urethral and vaginal suture lines by healthy tissue. *H*, if the vaginal mucosa does not provide an adequate covering or if it cannot be closed in a tension-free manner, a labial skin flap may be rotated as depicted. This provides full thickness cutaneous coverage and does not result in overlying urethral and cutaneous suture lines.

from a straddle injury. Their presentation and diagnosis is as described for the adult. The treatment involves placement of a small urethral catheter for partial tears. If the hematoma is large, it is drained. Complete tears require immediate repair as described for the adult or, if not

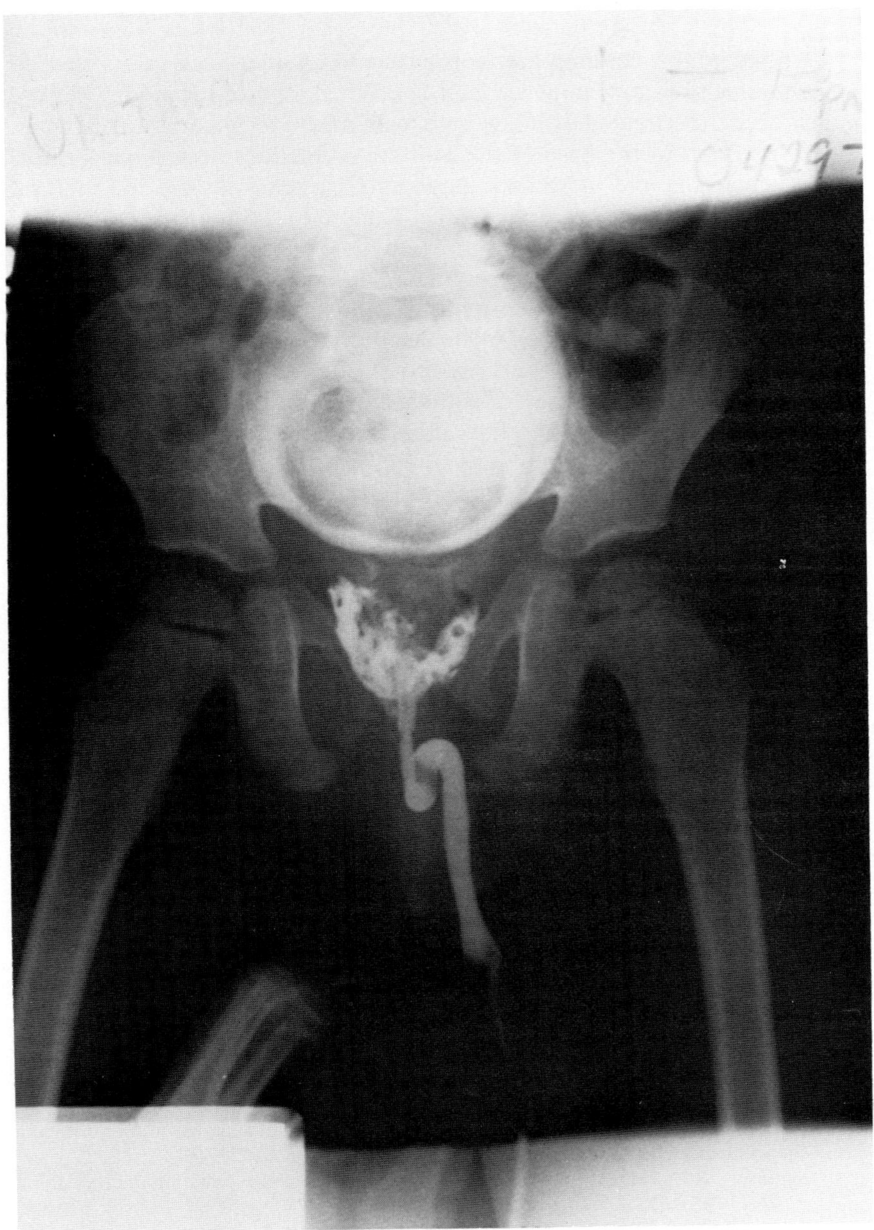

Figure 4.17. Traumatic prostatic urethral disruption in a child. The bladder is opacified by intravenous pyelographic dye and the urethra demonstrated by a retrograde urethrogram.

immediate, placement of a suprapubic catheter followed within 3 to 10 days by a primary repair.[19]

Posterior Urethra

Unlike adults, children are more prone to bladder neck injury than to prostatomembranous injury (Fig. 4.17). When a posterior urethral injury does occur, it is treated by immediate realignment over a urethral catheter. No dissection of the base of the prostate or bladder neck is performed. The hematoma and loose bone fragments are removed and the urethral catheter is tied to the suprapubic tube. The urethral catheter is maintained for 4 to 6 days on 200 to 400 g traction at 45° from the horizontal. The urogenital diaphragm must be intact, otherwise there is no support. Traction is removed and the urethral catheter is left in place for 4 to 6 weeks. Seven patients treated by this method had excellent results on long term follow-up. All were continent, potent, and voided well.[20] Complications are similar to those for adults; however, the development of a stricture in a child that requires more than one or two dilatations for definitive resolution should be repaired surgically since children tolerate repeated dilatations poorly. Care must always be exercised in choosing catheters for children. They should be of nonreactive material and must be small enough not to cause pressure necrosis or over distention of the urethra. A common sequela of indwelling catheters in children is stricture formation.

REFERENCES

1. Raney, A. M. Radiographic findings immediately after urethral rupture: an experimental study and case reports. *J. Urol. 116:*581, 1976.
2. Devine, C. J., Jr., Devine, P. C., and Horton, C. E. Anterior urethral injury: etiology, diagnosis, and initial management. *Urol. Clin. N. Amer. 4:*125, 1977.
3. Pontes, J. E., and Pierce, J. M., Jr. Anterior urethral injuries: four years of experience at the Detroit General Hospital. *J. Urol. 120:*563, 1978.
4. Turner-Warwick, R. A personal view of the immediate management of pelvic fracture urethral injuries. *Urol. Clin. N. Amer. 4:*81, 1977.
5. Weems, W. L. Management of genitourinary injuries in patients with pelvic fractures. *Ann. Surg. 189:*717, 1979.
6. Crassweller, P. O., Farrow, G. A., Robson, C. J., et al. Traumatic rupture of the supramembranous urethra. *J. Urol. 118:*770, 1977.
7. Colapinto, V., and McCallum, K. W. Injury to the male posterior urethra in fractured pelvis: a new classification. *J. Urol. 118:*575, 1977.
8. De Weerd, J. H. Immediate realignment of posterior urethral injury. *Urol. Clin. N. Amer. 4:*75, 1977.
9. Turner-Warwick, R. Observations on the treatment of traumatic urethral injuries and the value of the fenestrated urethral catheter. *Br. J. Surg. 60:*775, 1973.
10. Janknegt, R. A. Management of complete disruption of the posterior urethra. *Br. J. Urol. 47:*305, 1975.
11. Myers, R. P., and De Weerd, J. H. Incidence of stricture following primary realignment of the disrupted proximal urethra. *J. Urol. 107:*265, 1972.
12. Morehouse, D. D., Belitsky, P., and MacKinnon, K. Rupture of the posterior urethra. *J. Urol. 107:*255, 1972.
13. Waterhouse, R. K. Transpubic repair of membranous urethral strictures. *Urol. Clin. N. Amer. 4:*105, 1977.

TRAUMATIC INJURIES OF THE GENITOURINARY SYSTEM

14. Chatelain, C., LeGuillon, M., Petit, M., et al. Symphysiotomy or transpubic approach to traumatic strictures of the posterior urethra. *Eur. Urol. 1:*140, 1975.
15. Casselman, R. C., and Schillinger, J. F. Fractured pelvis with avulsion of the female urethra. *J. Urol. 117:*385, 1977.
16. Williams, D. I. Rupture of the female urethra in childhood. *Eur. Urol. 1:*129, 1975.
17. Morgan, J. E., Farrow, G. A., and Sims, R. H. The sloughed urethra syndrome. *Am. J. Obstet. Gynecol. 130:*521, 1978.
18. Simmends, K. E., and Hill, L. M. Loss of the urethra: a report on 50 patients. *Am. J. Obstet. Gynecol. 130:*130, 1978.
19. Garrett, R. A. Pediatric urethral and perineal injuries. *Ped. Clin. N. Amer. 22:*401, 1975.
20. Malels, R. S., O'Dea, M. J., and Kelales, P. P. Management of ruptured posterior urethra in childhood. *J. Urol. 117:*105, 1977.

5

Bladder Injuries

Bladder injuries occur as a result of blunt, penetrating, or operative trauma with males affected slightly more often than females. Irrespective of the type of trauma sustained, the injury is classified into one of four groups according to its extent and location in the bladder: 1) contusion, 2) extraperitoneal rupture, 3) intraperitoneal rupture, and 4) combined intraperitoneal and extraperitoneal rupture.

Blunt Trauma

Blunt trauma accounts for approximately 80% of all bladder injuries. Seventy percent of patients with blunt injuries to the bladder have an associated pelvic fracture; however, only 10 to 15% of patients with pelvic fractures sustain significant bladder injuries.[1] Extraperitoneal rupture is usually a consequence of a perforation sustained from a bony fragment; whereas, intraperitoneal ruptures invariably occur in the presence of a distended bladder.

A special case of blunt bladder injuries are those sustained during long distance running. Patients present with gross hematuria which clears rapidly—often after the first voiding. Slight suprapubic discomfort occurs inconsistently. The injury is a contusion which, when visualized cystoscopically, appears as hemorrhagic areas both at the base of the bladder and on the posterior wall. More severe injuries result in denudation of the mucosa followed by deposition of a fibrinous exudate. The injury occurs when the bladder is empty and appears to be due to the repeated impact of a flacid posterior wall on the bladder base.[2]

Obstetrical injuries may also result in bladder trauma. Pressure necrosis of the bladder base from prolonged pressure of the fetal head during a difficult delivery occurs occasionally. The injury is located at the trigone and bladder neck and is suspected when the patient either sloughs tissue in the urine or leaks urine per vagina on the third to fourteenth postpartum day. Rupture of the bladder is also seen concomitantly with spontaneous rupture of the gravid uterus.

85

Penetrating Injuries

These injuries occur as a consequence of a variety of weapons with the gun shot wound predominating. There is a slightly higher incidence of intraperitoneal injuries in penetrating trauma as compared to blunt trauma.

Operative Injuries

Operative injuries of the bladder are most commonly associated with obstetrical manipulations such as forceps deliveries and cesarian sections; gynecologic procedures such as suction D&C's, laparoscopy and pelvic surgery; and urologic manipulations requiring instrumentation of the lower urinary tract. Less common causes include perforation due to a Foley catheter which has remained indwelling for prolonged periods, orthopedic procedures of the hip and rectosigmoid resections.

SIGNS AND SYMPTOMS

Symptoms suggestive of bladder injury include inability to void, suprapubic pain, and incontinence. Lack of voiding is generally a result of the absence of urine in the bladder due to extravasation rather than outlet obstruction. Often the patients complain that they feel the need to void but cannot. Incontinence suggests a fistula; the most common type is a vesicovaginal fistula.

The most frequent presenting sign is hematuria which is present in the overwhelming majority of bladder injuries. A nonpalpable bladder may also suggest injury. Intraperitoneal extravasation of urine may result in abdominal ileus and distension; however, providing the urine is sterile, it is surprisingly well tolerated and often produces no symptoms. Indeed, there are patients who have consumed large quantities of alcohol and subsequently sustained blunt trauma to a distended bladder with resultant intraperitoneal rupture who after several days complain only of the inability to void. Vital signs are often stable and at exploration there is often very little if any intraperitoneal reaction.[3] If the urine is infected, however, frank peritonitis supervenes.

DIAGNOSIS

Early diagnosis is important for significant delays greatly increase morbidity and mortality.[4] The definitive diagnosis is made by cystography when a rupture is present and by cystoscopy when a contusion has been sustained. The cystogram is performed by inserting a Foley catheter into the bladder (urethral injuries must be excluded before the bladder is catheterized—see Chapter 4) and allowing it to fill by gravity with 300 to 400 cc of radiocontrast. An anterior-posterior view, obliques, and post-evacuation films are obtained. The postevacuation film is essential in order to exclude small posterior or anterior perforations which may be hidden by the dye-distended bladder. It is performed by allowing the

     TRAUMATIC INJURIES OF THE GENITOURINARY SYSTEM

contrast to flow out of the bladder followed by the instillation of 50 cc of saline. The saline is allowed to drain out, thus washing any residual dye from the intravesicle portion of the bladder. If time is of the essence and only a limited number of films can be obtained, the most important roentgenograms are the anterior-posterior view of the distended bladder and the postevacuation film. Extraperitoneal rupture is indicated by the extravasated dye remaining in the confines of the low pelvis (Fig. 5.1). An intraperitoneal rupture is suggested when the dye outlines loops of bowel or is visualized along the lateral gutters (Fig. 5.2).

Contusions are suspected when the trauma has been sustained to the region of the bladder, hematuria is present, and the cystogram reveals no extravasation. The diagnosis is established cystoscopically; however, this is usually unnecessary since the clinical signs are sufficiently suggestive. Moreover, cystoscopy rarely alters treatment. The cystoscopic appearance reveals ecchymoses, focal areas of hemorrhage, or localized areas where the mucosa has been denuded. A fibrinous exudate overlying the hemorrhagic areas may be observed later in the patient's course.

TREATMENT

Contusions

Contusions are treated nonoperatively. If the patient is able to void spontaneously, a catheter is not required; however, often the extent of trauma makes voiding difficult and a catheter is inserted for the patient's convenience. If a Foley catheter is left indwelling, it should be connected to a closed tube drainage system. Patients with indwelling catheters and those with pre-existing urinary tract infections are treated with prophylactic antibiotics.

Extraperitoneal Rupture

There is some controversy regarding the treatment of these injuries. They may be managed either conservatively or by operative repair. There are several reports of successful management of these lesions by urethral catheter drainage, antibiotics, and observation.[5, 6] The catheter remains in place for 1 to 5 weeks and a cystogram must be performed prior to its removal to confirm bladder integrity. Patients who may be considered for conservative management are 1) those who do not have an antecedent urinary tract infection, 2) patients in whom the rupture is recognized within several hours of injury, and 3) those who have small tears which are not multiple.

Surgical therapy is preferred by many for all ruptures of the bladder; however, it is mandatory when the injury is extensive. The bladder is opened, the rents debrided, and sutured with chromic catgut suture and a suprapubic cystostomy placed. The perivesicle space is drained and the patient placed on antibiotics. Proponents of this management point out that those in whom the bladder lesion contributes significantly to mortality are patients who either have not had a suprapubic tube placed when operated upon or have been treated nonoperatively.[4] Our policy is to

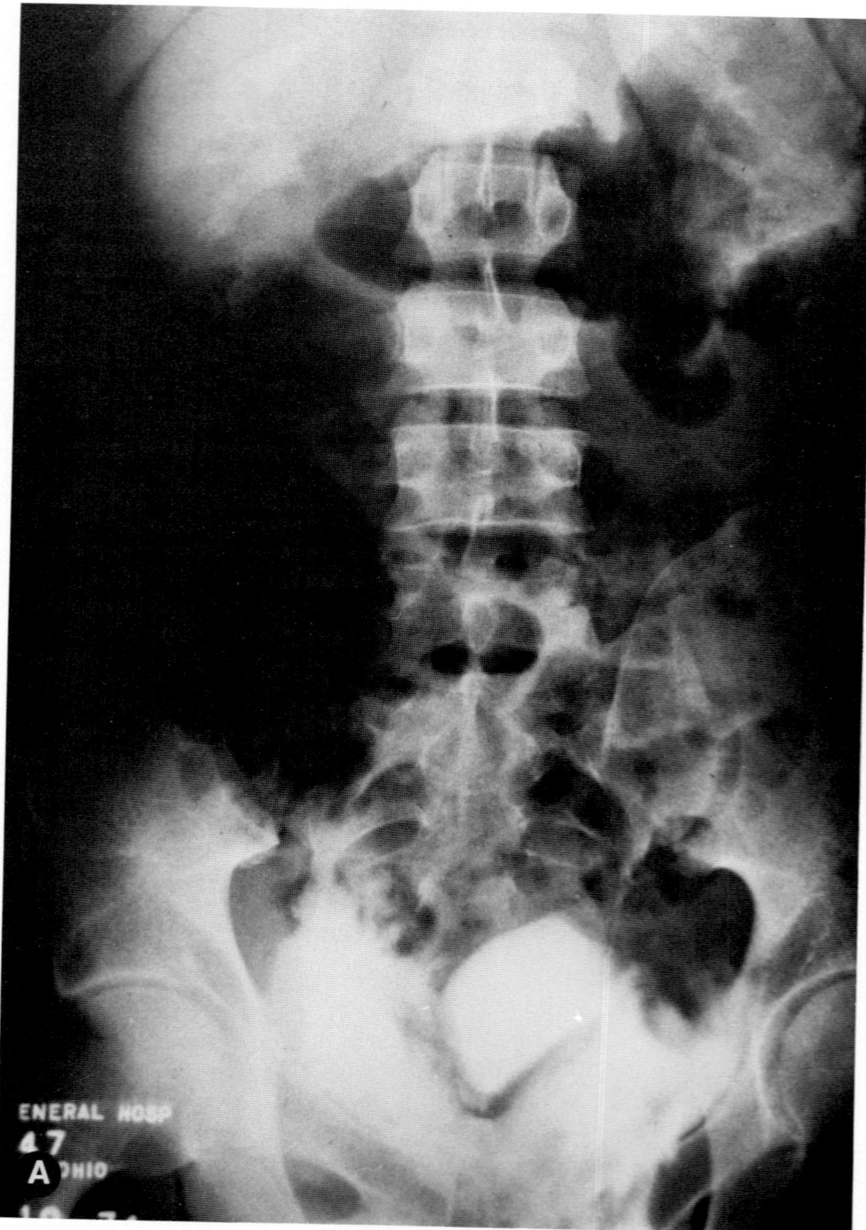

Figure 5.1. Intravenous pyelograms of extraperitoneal bladder rupture due to blunt trauma (*A*) and penetrating trauma (*B*).

explore all patients with a ruptured bladder unless the extraperitoneal extravasation is of limited extent and the other criteria described above are met.

Intraperitoneal Rupture

Similarly, conservative and operative management have been advocated for these lesions. Providing the patient has uninfected urine, the

TRAUMATIC INJURIES OF THE GENITOURINARY SYSTEM

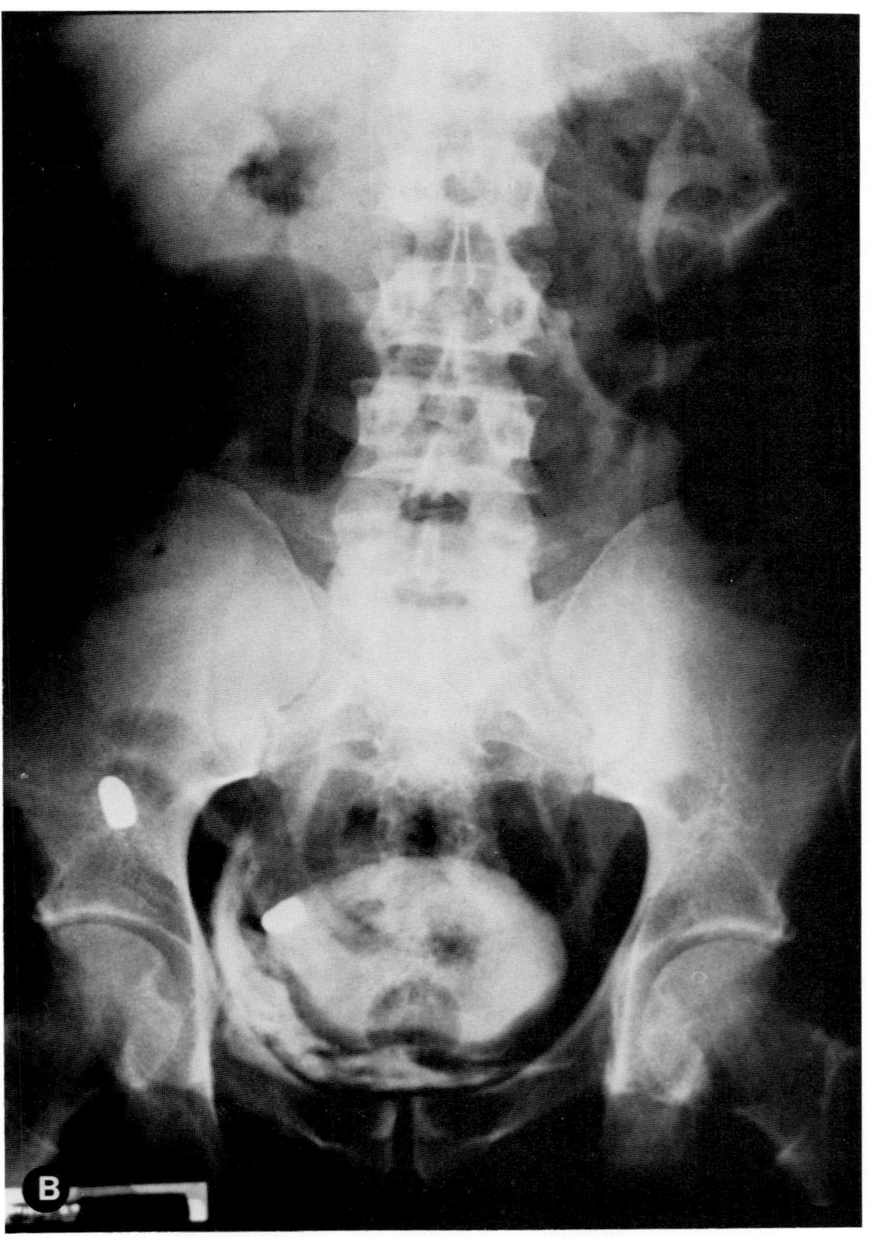

injury is recognized within several hours of occurence, and a large caliber catheter can be easily inserted, success has been reported using catheter drainage, prophylactic antibiotics, and observation.[5] However, it is our preference to operate and repair all intraperitoneal ruptures since morbidity is significantly reduced. Although no prospective study has been performed, it appears that mortality is also reduced when intraperitoneal ruptures are managed by operative intervention.

BLADDER INJURIES   89

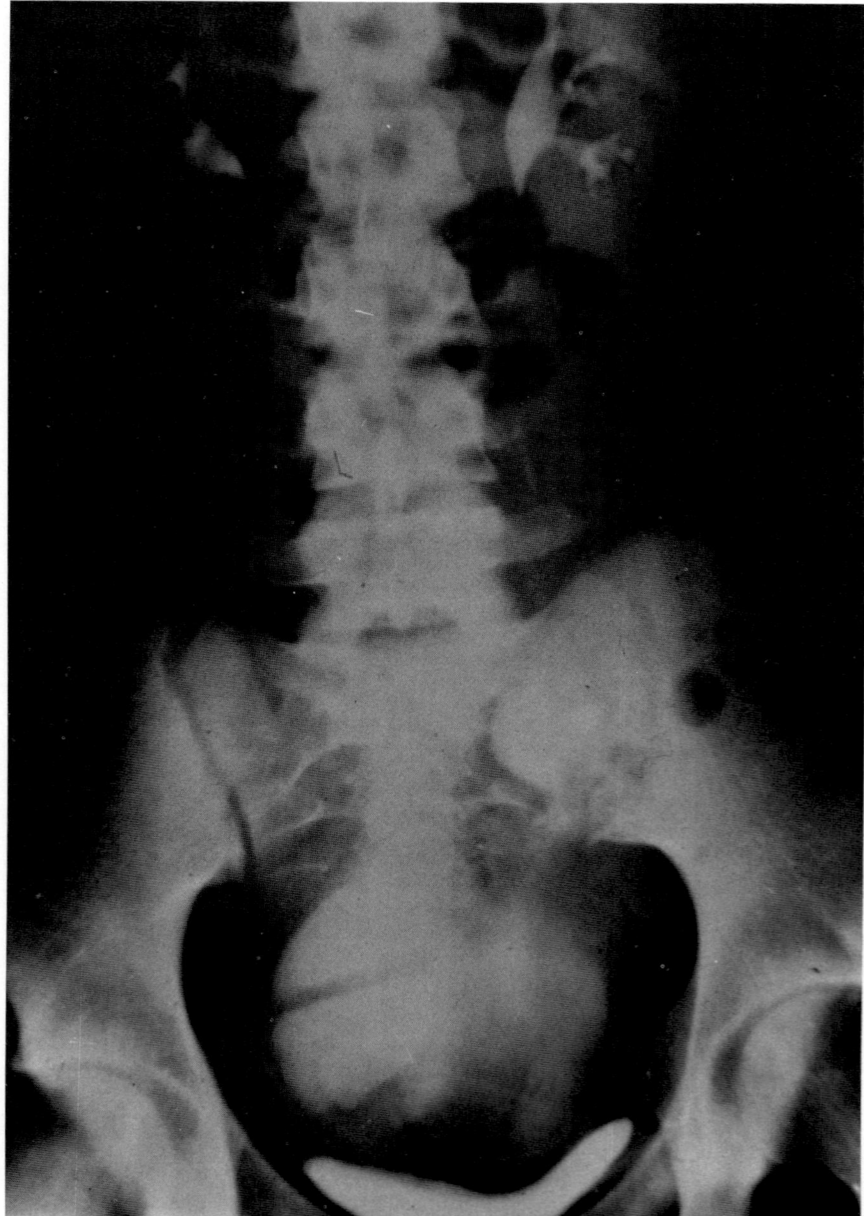

Figure 5.2. Intravenous pyelogram of intraperitoneal bladder rupture. Notice the bowel outlined by the dye.

MORTALITY

Bladder injuries are rarely lethal in and of themselves. Patients who sustain trauma to the bladder often have significant associated injuries, and it is from these that the patient usually succumbs. The mortality

     TRAUMATIC INJURIES OF THE GENITOURINARY SYSTEM

varies between 11 and 31% in patients who have multiple injuries in addition to vesicle rupture.[4] Although often not directly responsible for a patient's demise, bladder injuries contribute significantly to morbidity. If not recognized early, not only do they increase morbidity but they increase mortality as well.

COMPLICATIONS

Cystitis and chronic urinary tract infections are the most common complications. They may be minimized by aseptic insertion of the catheter and maintenance of a closed tube drainage system. Infections of the retropubic space may be found following an operative procedure on the bladder, but do occur on occasion in patients with extravasation who are treated conservatively. Periureteral fibrosis occurs as a consequence of urinary extravasation and may cause ureteral obstruction.[7] Finally, vesicovaginal fistulae occur most frequently following gynecologic and obstetric procedures. They have also been seen as a consequence of blunt perineal trauma.

Vesicovaginal Fistula Repair

Many methods of treating vesicovaginal fistulae have been advocated and include catheter and/or postural drainage, cauterization, and surgical repair either by the transvaginal or transabdominal approach. On rare occasion, when the fistula is small and located on the fixed portion of the bladder (trigone), catheter drainage may result in a successful outcome; however, if the injury is located elsewhere in the bladder, prolonged catheter drainage generally has little effect. Cauterization is rarely if ever useful in traumatic injuries as a method of repair. Surgical repair is generally the procedure of choice and should be performed as soon as the acute inflammatory process subsides and the fistula matures. We generally prefer to approach the injury transabdominally. The vagina is packed preoperatively and antibiotics are administered. The bladder is dissected from the vagina, the edges of the vaginal defect are debrided, and the wound closed with resorbable sutures. The fistula walls in the bladder are excised being careful not to injure the ureters. On occasion, proper excision and closure requires ureteral reimplantation. The bladder is closed in layers with interrupted resorbable sutures: the mucosa from the inside through a cystotomy and the muscularis from outside the bladder. The vaginal and bladder suture lines must be separated by either a pedicle of peritoneum formed from that which covers the cephalad wall of the bladder or by an omental pedicle flap (see Chapter 4). The latter provides a more secure buffer between the two suture lines.

BLADDER INJURIES IN CHILDREN

The bladder of a child is more of an intra-abdominal organ than that of an adult and is therefore less well protected by the bony pelvis. Bladder

injuries which occur as a consequence of violent blunt trauma are almost
always associated with pelvic fractures. Other causes unique to the child
include rupture as a consequence of crede maneuver, laceration during
an umbilical artery cutdown due to the bladder's intra-abdominal position
and proximity to the umbilicus, and rupture of a congenital diverticulum.
Often the patients develop urinary ascites as the rupture is intraperitoneal.[8] Operative intervention is indicated with repair and drainage. Unfortunately, there appears to be a greater incidence of infection of the
space of Retzius postoperatively in children than occurs following operative therapy of bladder injuries in adults.[9]

REFERENCES

1. Brasman, S. A., and Paul, J. G. Trauma of the bladder. *Surg. Gynecol. Obstet. 143:*605, 1976.
2. Blacklock, N. J. Bladder trauma in the long-distance runner: "10,000 metres haematuria." *Br. J. Med. 49:*129, 1977.
3. Carswell, J. W. Intraperitoneal rupture of the bladder. *Br. J. Urol. 46:*425, 1974.
4. Cass, A. S. Bladder trauma in the multiple injuried patient. *J. Urol. 115:*667, 1976.
5. Robards, V. L., Haglund, R. V., Lubin, E. W., et al. Treatment of rupture of the bladder. *J. Urol. 116:*178, 1976.
6. Richardson, J. R., Jr., and Leadbetter, G. W., Jr. Non-operative treatment of the ruptured bladder. *J. Urol. 114:*213, 1975.
7. Rao, M. S., Bapna, B. C., and Vaidyanathan, S. Ureteral and periureteral fibrosis as delayed sequelae to lower urinary tract injury. *J. Urol. 113:*610, 1975.
8. Redman, J. F., Seibert, J. J., and Watson, A. Urinary ascites in children owing to extravasation of urine from the bladder. *J. Urol. 122:*409, 1979.
9. Sinclair, M. C., Moore, T. C., Asch, M. J., et al. Injury to hollow abdominal viscera from blunt trauma in children and adolescents. *Am. J. Surg. 128:*693, 1974.

6

Ureteral Injuries

Traumatic ureteral injuries are the result of either blunt trauma, penetrating trauma, or operative misadventure. Irrespective of etiology, they are uncommon injuries accounting for less than one-tenth of 1% of all surgical hospital patients. Indeed, only 2.3% of patients who sustain gun shot wounds to the abdomen have ureteral involvement.[1] The rarity of the lesion may be accounted for by the flexibility of the ureter, its small size, and the protection afforded by the muscular and bony structures which surround it.

ETIOLOGY

Penetrating Trauma

Penetrating trauma accounts for more than 90% of the nonoperative injuries. Bullets, knives, and shrapnel are the usual agents. The damage they cause is dependent upon their velocity at the time of impact. The extent of tissue injury in low velocity wounds is generally easily appreciated visually by the surgeon, whereas the damage high velocity wounds inflict is often not immediately apparent. High velocity injuries occur when the missle travels at a speed greater than 2500 feet per second. At impact rapid expansion and compression of surrounding tissues results in their damage. The extent of damage caused by this concussion is directly proportional to the mass of the missle and the square of its velocity. Therefore, the velocity of the missle bears directly on the surgical therapy. High velocity wounds require extensive debridement to bleeding tissue, whereas low velocity injuries require a less extensive debridement in order to gain freely bleeding wound margins.

Blunt Trauma

Blunt trauma is an infrequent cause of ureteral injuries. A bony spicule from a fractured transverse process or vertebral body or acute hyperextension in which tension is placed upon the ureter are the usual mecha-

93

nisms. In children, particularly young boys, disruption of the ureteropelvic junction is the injury most commonly found as a result of hyperextension.

Operative Injuries

Operative or iatrogenic injuries are most commonly associated with gynecologic procedures (Fig. 6.1). The proximity of the ureter to the cervix and uterine arteries makes it particularly vulnerable. Other procedures in which injuries of the ureter occur include rectal excision, aortic surgery, sigmoid and colon resections, excision of retroperitoneal masses or lymph nodes, dissections in the presence of retroperitoneal fibrosis, sympathectomy, laminectomy, and pancreatic and duodenal manipulations. Urologic procedures commonly responsible for injury include retrograde catheter placement and stone basket manipulation.

ASSOCIATED INJURIES

Significant associated injuries are frequently encountered when the ureteral injury is a consequence of a gun shot wound. Those structures most commonly injured in descending order of occurrance are the small bowel, colon, liver, pancreas, bladder, duodenum, rectum, and great vessels. Indeed, the iliac vein was injured in 6 of 11 patients who sustained a gun shot wound to the midureter.[2] Blunt traumatic ureteral injuries are invariably associated with bony fractures and/or renal, bladder and visceral organ fractures or contusions.

SIGNS AND SYMPTOMS

Unfortunately, many ureteral injuries are not recognized initially or even early during their course. This is in part due to the rarity of the lesion and, therefore, the lack of its inclusion in the differential diagnosis. The fact that the injury almost never presents as an isolated lesion also complicates the situation. Moreover, associated injuries often take precedence in the critically ill trauma patient and normal postoperative pain in patients who have sustained operative injuries often make the diagnosis difficult. Hematuria occurs in 70 to 90% of patients with penetrating injuries; however, it is present in only 10% of those who have sustained an operative injury.[3, 4] Flank pain, abdominal discomfort, ileus, anuria, sepsis, and hyperchloremic acidosis suggest the diagnosis. Urinary fistulae and urinary tract infections occur later in the course.

DIAGNOSIS

Early diagnosis and immediate therapy lessen morbidity and result in maximal preservation of renal parenchyma.[5] Moreover, delayed recognition in the patient who sustains a nonoperative injury results in a much poorer prognosis than delay in recognizing an operative injury.[6] There-

TRAUMATIC INJURIES OF THE GENITOURINARY SYSTEM

fore, a high index of suspicion is critical for proper patient management. Urine analysis combined with infusion pyelography is diagnostic in more than 90% of the cases (Fig. 6.2). In selected patients where the diagnosis is in doubt, retrograde pyelography confirms the location and extent of injury. Operative injuries may be diagnosed by performing an intraoperative intravenous pyelogram or by the intravenous administration of 5 to 10 cc of indigo carmen. The injury is located by the appearance of blue dye in the wound. Indigo carmen may be combined with a 12.5 g mannitol infusion in the hemodynamically stable patient to increase the volume of blue fluid issuing from the injured site and thereby improve diagnostic accuracy. Ultrasonography is helpful in patients who have sustained operative injuries in which the ureter is obstructed. If the sonogram demonstrates hydronephrosis, the need for further studies are suggested to confirm the diagnosis.

TREATMENT

Prompt recognition of ureteral injuries and immediate surgical repair result in an increased incidence of renal units preserved, a decreased incidence of ureteral complications requiring a second procedure, and reduced morbidity when compared to patients in whom a delayed repair is performed. Although an immediate surgical approach is indicated in most instances, there are exceptions. In selected patients, observation may be all that is required. Minor injuries such as those sustained as a result of a ureteral catheter perforation may be treated nonoperatively (Fig. 6.3), provided the ureteral defect is small, there is no distal obstruction, there are no associated injuries, the ureter is not diseased, and ureteral continuity is maintained.[7] Patients in whom the injury is recognized later in the post-traumatic course during a period of instability or in the presence of a periureteral abscess or severe inflammation may require a temporary diversion with the primary repair delayed until the periureteral inflammatory process has resolved and the patient is stable. The diversion may be accomplished by a percutaneous or open nephrostomy. The former may be performed at the bedside if necessary under sonographic control.

There are a number of surgical procedures which have been employed to treat ureteral injuries and include ureteroureterostomy, tube ureterostomy, intentional ligation, deligation, ureteroneocystostomy with or without a psoas bladder hitch or Boari pedicle flap, transureteroureterostomy, ileal substitution, and autotransplantation. Each procedure is indicated for specific types of injuries; however, there are basic principles which are common to each of the procedures. The injured area must be adequately debrided. All nonviable tissue must be removed and that which remains must freely bleed from its cut edges. The ureter must be adequately mobilized, being careful to preserve its blood supply which comes to it from a medial direction. The ureter is adequately mobilized when the debrided ends may be brought together without tension. A spatulated water tight anastomosis with interrupted atraumatic 4-0 chromic catgut

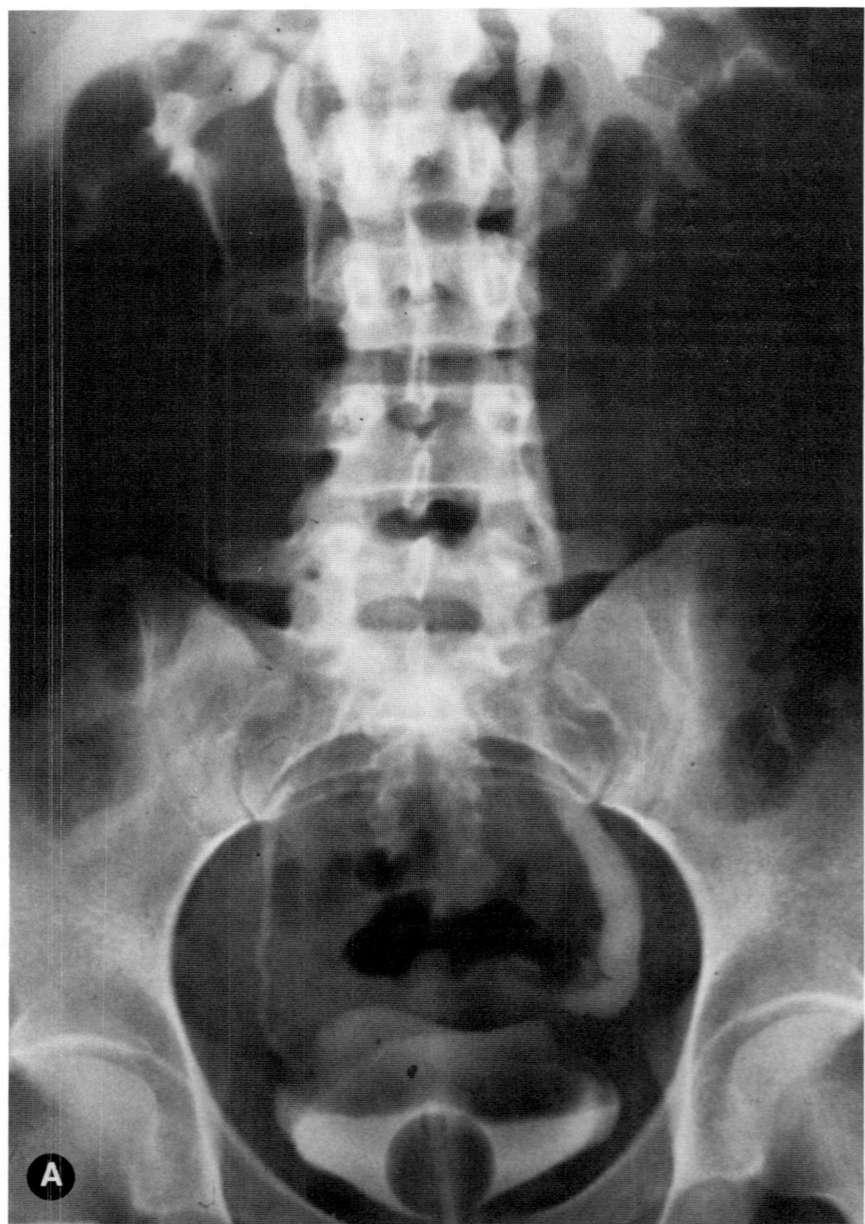

Figure 6.1. Ureterovaginal fistula following an abdominal hysterectomy. *A*, intravenous pyelogram demonstrating a left hydroureteronephrosis with extravasation of dye into the vagina. *B*, lateral view of the intravenous pyelogram illustrating the distal left ureter and dye filled vagina.

sutures must be performed. The anastomosis must be drained retroperitoneally. The drains must serve to drain only the injured ureter and should be excluded from other injured organs, particularly the duodenum and the pancreas. The anastomosis should be surrounded by retroperito-

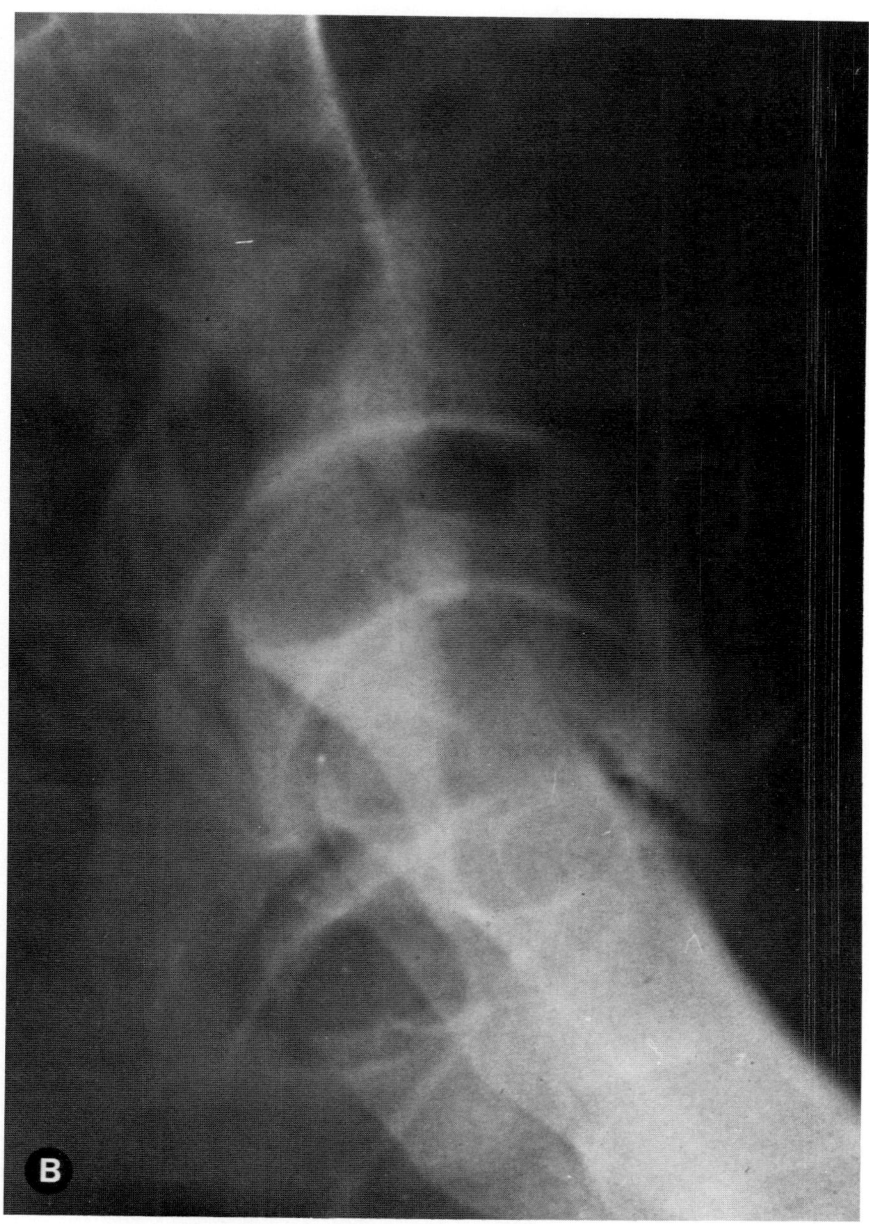

neal fat or an omental pedicle (the creation of an omental pedicle is described in Chapter 4). Finally, antibiotics are administered and infection controlled.

Ureteroureterostomy

This procedure is indicated for limited injuries of the mid and upper ureter. After proper debridement, the defect can be no greater than that

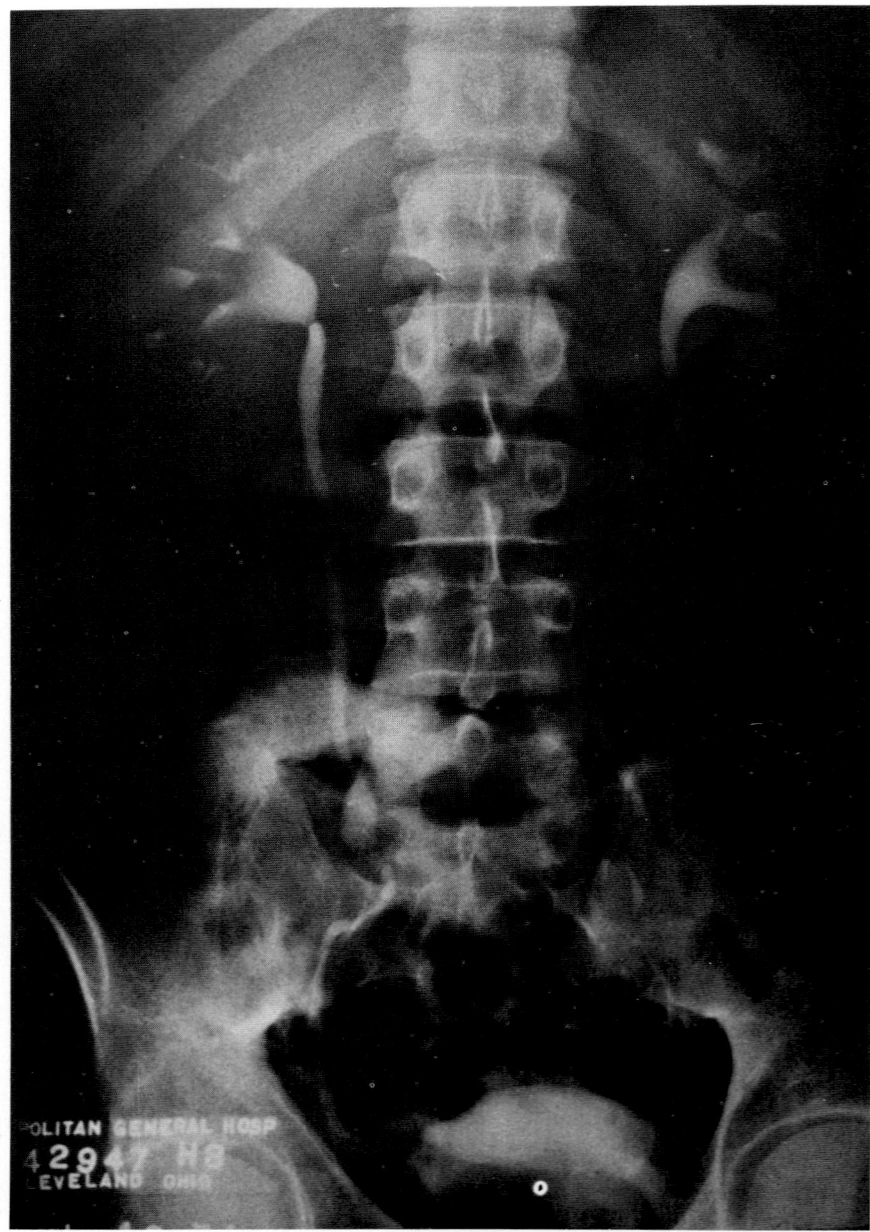

Figure 6.2. Intravenous pyelogram in a patient who sustained a right ureteral injury as a result of a gun shot wound. Notice the extravasated dye to the right of L4 and L5.

which will allow for a tension-free anastomosis. The cut ends of the ureter are spatulated, 180° from each other and sewn together with interrupted 4-0 chromic catgut suture so that a water tight seal is obtained (Fig. 6.4). A water tight anastomosis is critical for a successful outcome. A nonwater tight anastomosis results in a 20 to 50% incidence of postoperative

     TRAUMATIC INJURIES OF THE GENITOURINARY SYSTEM

stricture, whereas a water tight suture line results in a very small rate of stricture formation.[1, 4] The suture line can be checked for its integrity by occluding the ureter below and infusing saline above. The anastomosis should be surrounded with retroperitoneal fat or an omental pedicle flap. The latter has the advantage of providing a flexible supportive structure which maintains pliability of the ureter, defends against infection, and provides increased blood flow to the area.

The use of stents is a subject of controversy. The advantages of their use include diversion of urine away from the anastomosis, thereby reducing reactive fibrous tissue formation secondary to urinary extravasation and providing a scaffold about which the ureter may heal. The disadvantage of their use, however, is that stricture formation may be promoted if the stent irritates the anastomosis. Stents must be used when the anastomosis is under tension, there is evidence of ureteral ischemia or infection, or a concomitant pancreatic, duodenal, or major vascular injury has been sustained. In the presence of associated pancreatic, duodenal, and major vascular injuries, a nephrostomy is performed in addition to the placement of a ureteral stent. A urine leak in patients with these associated injuries results in an exceedingly high mortality rate.[8, 9] Proponents of the stent suggest that there are fewer postoperative complications with their routine use.[10] Irrespective of the type of stent employed, it must be large enough to completely divert the urine yet not so large as to place pressure on the anastomosis. The stent must also be fixed in place so that it does not become inadvertly dislodged in the immediate postoperative period. It is left in place for 2 to 3 weeks and when removed, injected with dye under fluoroscopy so that the integrity of the anastomosis may be confirmed.

A number 8 pediatric feeding tube or similar sized polyethylene tube placed from renal pelvis to bladder serves satisfactorily. One end must be secured so that the tube does not dislodge. The distal end may be secured to a catheter which may be brought out either suprapubically or via the urethra; or the proximal end may be brought out along side a nephrostomy tube. Alternatively, a T tube may be placed through a vertical ureterotomy either above or below the anastomosis with one side arm positioned so that the suture line is stented. Prior to the insertion of the T tube, a wedge of rubber is cut away from the junction of the T at its base, which allows for a less traumatic removal postoperatively.

If the anastomosis is tension-free and water tight, there is no surrounding infection, and significant associated injuries are not present, it may be left unstented. A proximal ureterotomy is performed and both the anastomosis and ureterotomy drained separately. In properly selected patients, this technique results in a very low incidence of postoperative ureteral complications.[4]

Tube Ureterostomy

Patients who are unstable at the time of surgery and in whom operative time must be curtailed may benefit from a temporizing procedure which can be expiditiously performed such as tube ureterostomy (Fig. 6.5). The tube must be secured to the skin as well as the ureter and provides for

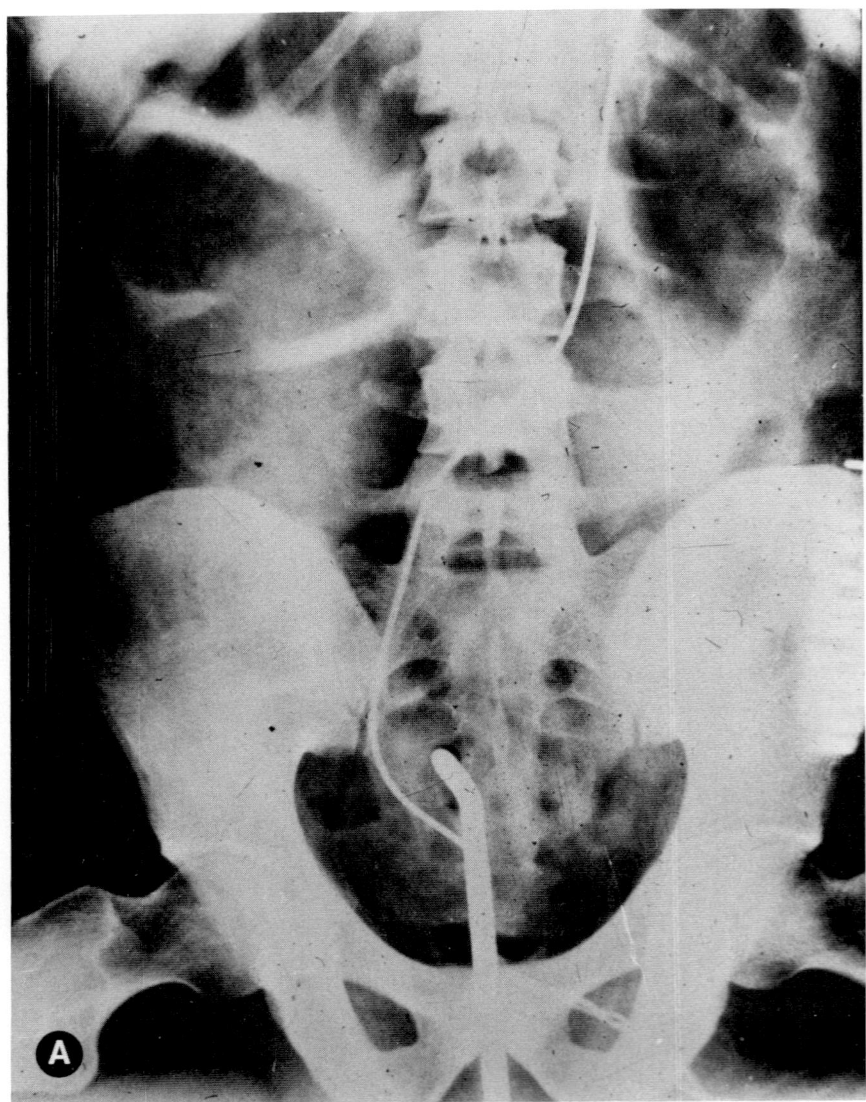

Figure 6.3. Perforation of the ureter by a retrograde catheter. *A*, the retrograde catheter has perforated the distal right ureter and passed to the opposite side of the abdomen. The catheter was removed and the patient observed. An intravenous pyelogram obtained 1 month postinjury demonstrates a normal collecting system on the right (*B*).

drainage of the renal unit until a more definitive procedure can be performed. The ureter should not be extensively dissected. Unfortunately, tube ureterostomies have a way of "falling out" in the postoperative period no matter how well secured and should be used only when there is no other acceptable alternative. A second operation to restore ureteral continuity is required at a later date.

     TRAUMATIC INJURIES OF THE GENITOURINARY SYSTEM

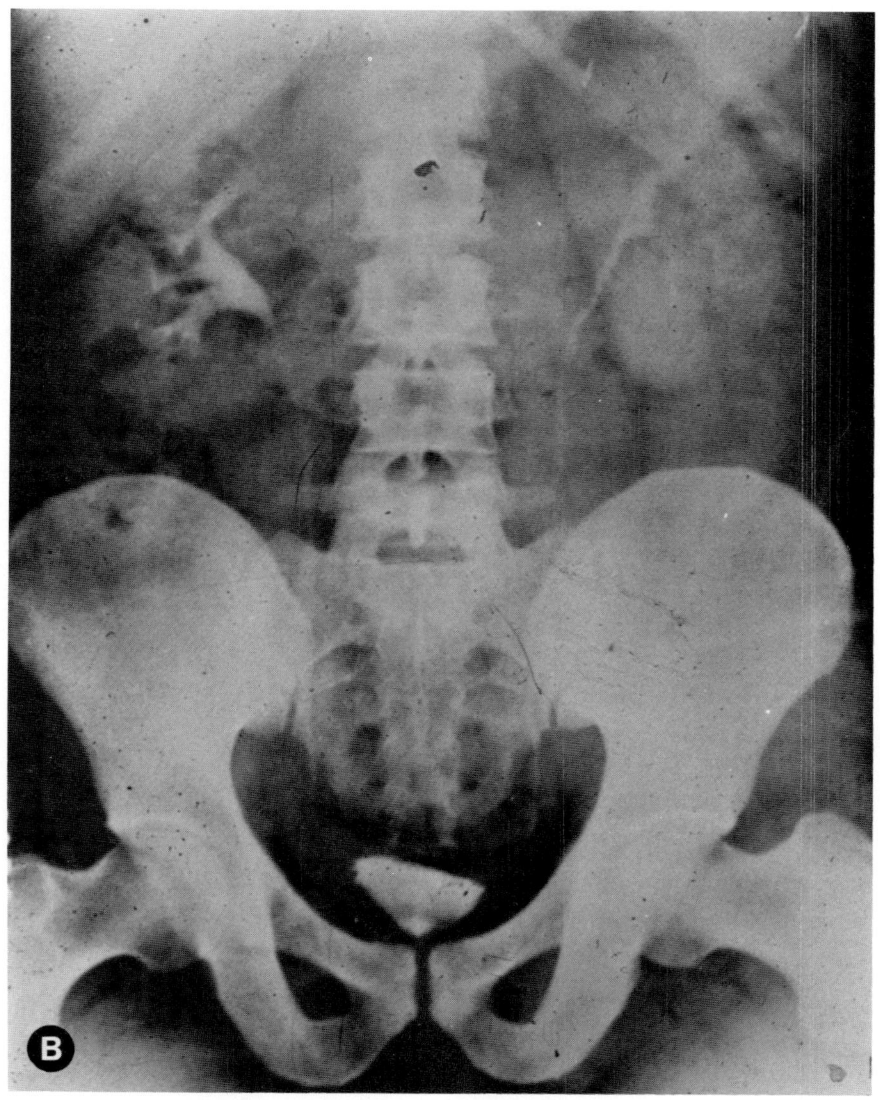

Intentional Ureteral Ligation

This procedure is to be condemned, particularly in the critically ill traumatized patient. It results in a considerable incidence of fistulae and sepsis and adds greatly to the postinjury morbidity.

Deligation

Ligatures may be inadvertantly placed about the ureter during an operative procedure. If recognized intraoperatively, simple deligation will suffice provided the ureter is viable. Ligatures which are recognized

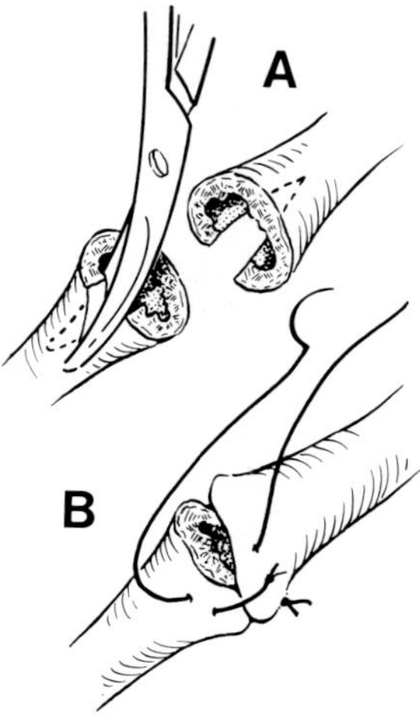

Figure 6.4. Spatulated ureteral anastomosis. Notice that the spatulation on one end is made on the opposite side from that of the other.

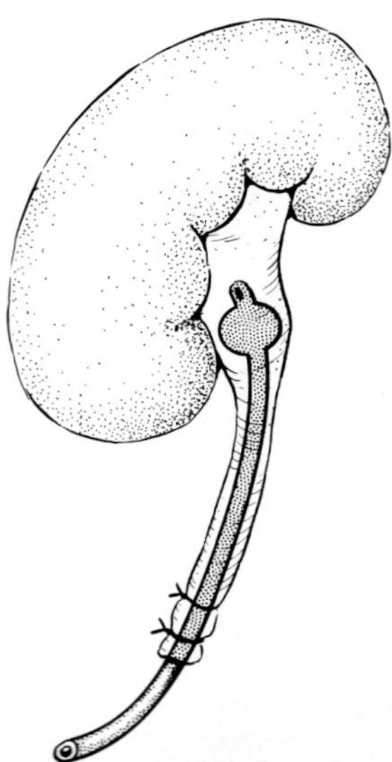

Figure 6.5. Tube ureterostomy. The indwelling tube is secured to both the ureter and the skin and the area drained.

postoperatively and are occlusive should be removed as soon as they are discovered (Fig. 6.6). It has been demonstrated experimentally that simple deligation may be performed up to 1 week after ligature placement without complications. If removed between 1 and 2 weeks without ureteral reconstruction, a successful outcome may be anticipated in 50% of the cases. Ligatures which are in place for more than 2 weeks prior to removal invariably result in a ureteral stricture. Moreover, resorbable sutures left in situ with the hope that they will dissolve result in significant permanent damage to the renal unit.[11] Ureters in which the suture has been in place for more than 1 week or those which appear stenotic after the suture is

     TRAUMATIC INJURIES OF THE GENITOURINARY SYSTEM

removed, require ureteral calibration. A proximal ureterotomy allows passage of graded catheters. If the ureteral wall is nonviable or stenotic, a ureteroureterostomy is performed.

Ureteroneocystostomy

Whenever possible, a ureteroneocystostomy is the procedure of choice for lower ureteral injuries since it provides the least complication rate and morbidity. The anastomosis must be tension-free and nonrefluxing. In our hands, reimplantation by a modification of the Politano-Leadbetter procedure has provided the best results (Fig. 6.7). Lower ureteral injuries which cannot be reimplanted without tension require a bladder extension procedure. With the psoas bladder hitch or a psoas bladder hitch combined with a Boari pedicle flap, defects as high as L-4,5 can be bridged. The psoas hitch is performed by mobilizing the bladder and securing it to the psoas minor tendon (or psoas major when the minor is congenitally absent). The contralateral superior vesicle artery must be ligated and severed and the surrounding tissue freed from the bladder in order to gain adequate mobility (Fig. 6.8). The Boari procedure is performed by creating a pedicle flap whose base is cephalad and includes the superior vesicle artery on the same side. A tube is created and the ureter placed beneath a submucosal tunnel in the end of the tube (Fig. 6.9). A common late complication encountered is stricture of the Boari pedicle tube. This is more likely to occur if the base and width of the tube are made too small.

Transureteroureterostomy

This procedure is almost never indicated in the traumatized patient at the time of initial exploration and should never be employed in patients in whom there is a history of calculus disease, retroperitoneal fibrosis, tuberculosis, transitional cell carcinoma of the upper urinary tract, or obstruction or disease of the recipient ureter. It may be used when the injury is located below the pelvis. The recipient ureter is mobilized as little as possible and the injured ureter brought beneath the mesentary cephalad to the inferior mesenteric artery, spatulated and sutured obliquely into the recipient ureter (Fig. 6.10). The disadvantage of the procedure is that should anastomotic complications occur, both renal units are affected.

Ileal Substitution

When long segments of ureter are damaged and the defect cannot be bridged by one of the procedures previously described, a segment of small bowel may be used to restore continuity. The kidney is completely mobilized and pexed caudally. The bladder is mobilized and a psoas hitch performed as previously described. This allows for the shortest possible bowel segment. An ileal segment is isolated and a rent made in the mesocolon. The ileal segment is placed in the retroperitoneum and the proximal portion sutured to the renal pelvis. On occasion, the pyelostomy

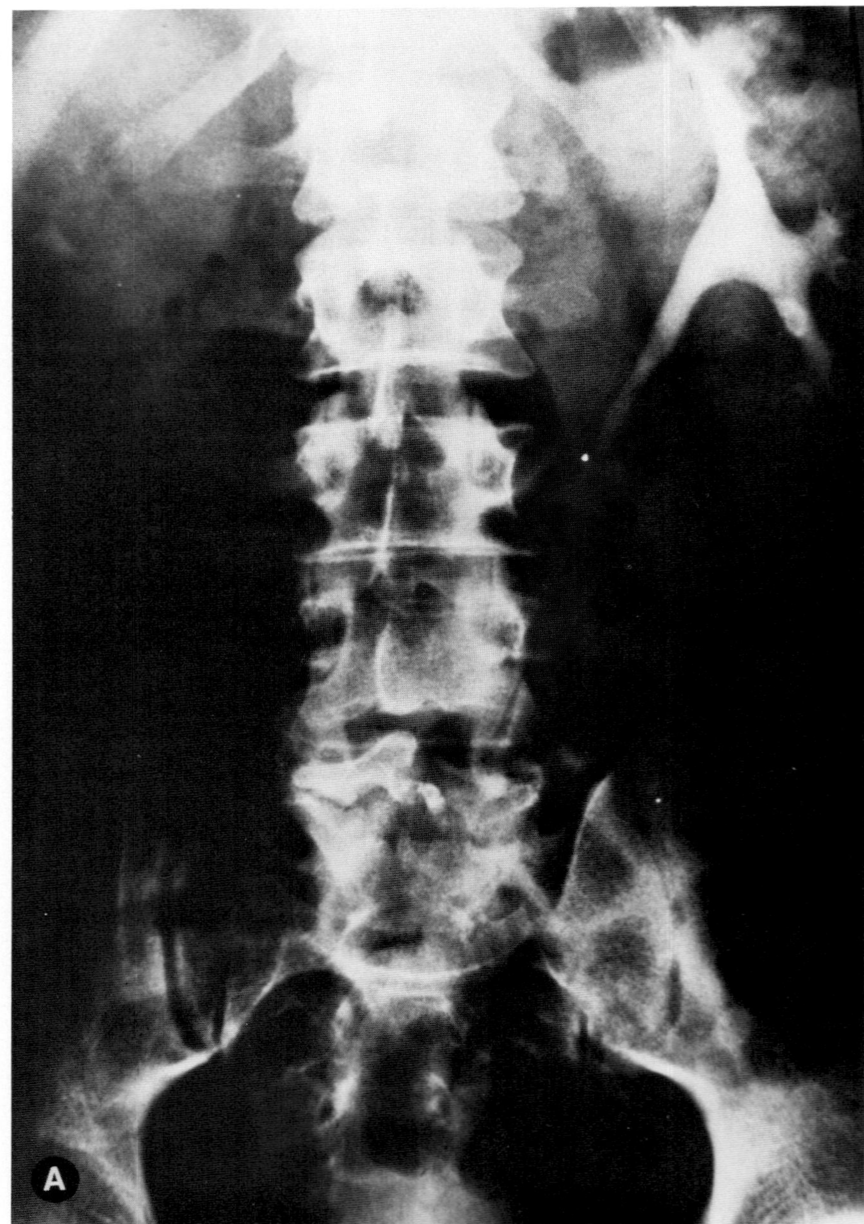

Figure 6.6. Inadvertant ligation of the distal right ureter during the removal of an ovarian cyst. *A*, intravenous pyelogram 2 days postoperative demonstrating nonvisualization of the right collecting system. *B*, retrograde pyelogram illustrating the ligature about the distal ureter.

must be extended into the inferior calyx to provide for adequate drainage. A nephrostomy is placed and a stent placed through the segment and brought out with the nephrostomy. The distal portion of the ileal segment is sutured to the bladder (Fig. 6.11).

     TRAUMATIC INJURIES OF THE GENITOURINARY SYSTEM

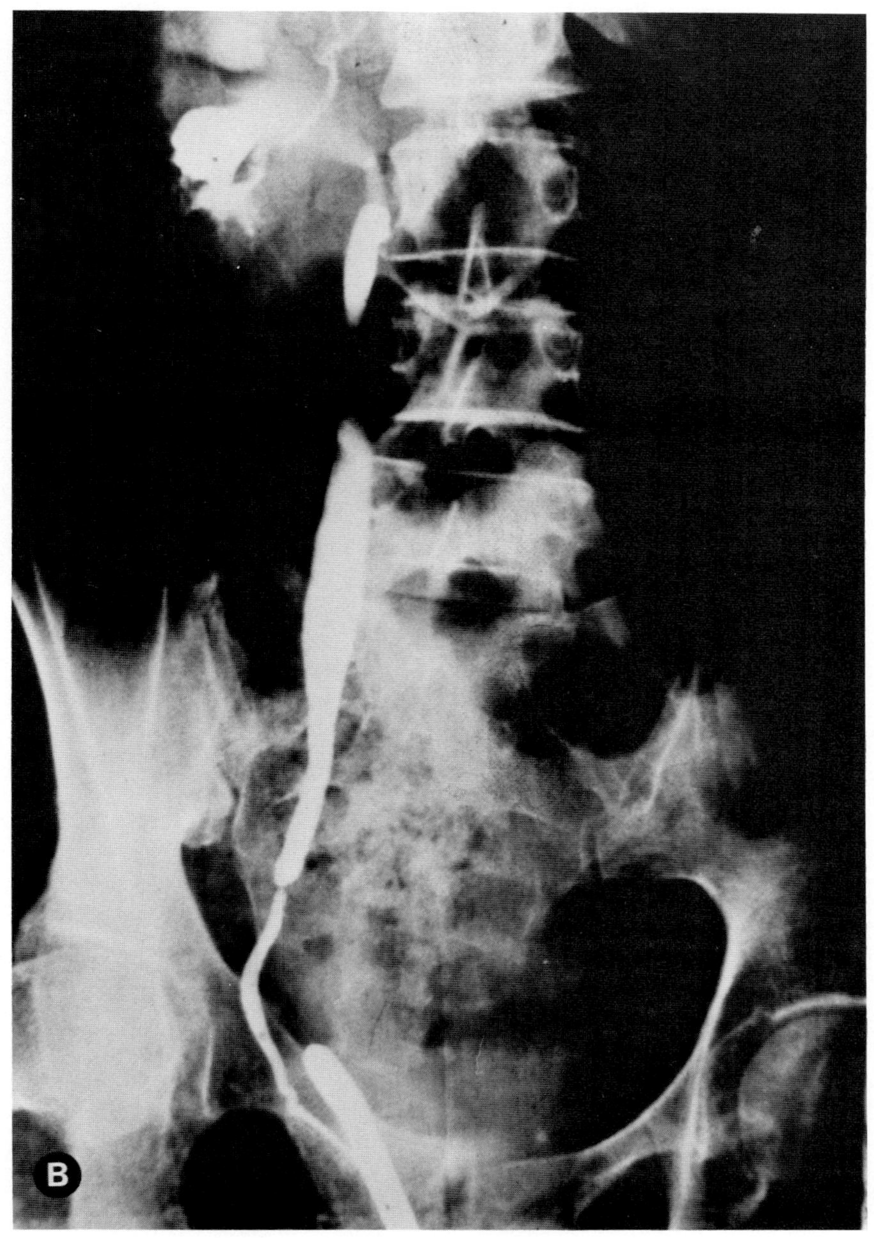

The bowel continues to secrete mucus which is voided by the patient. The mucus may cause symptoms of outlet obstruction, particularly in males, and bladder neck revision may be required in order to establish uninhibited voiding. These patients must be followed carefully for if they develop significant outlet obstruction, be it due to mucus or prostatism, the bowel segment dilates, becomes atonic, and drains the kidney poorly.

URETERAL INJURIES 105

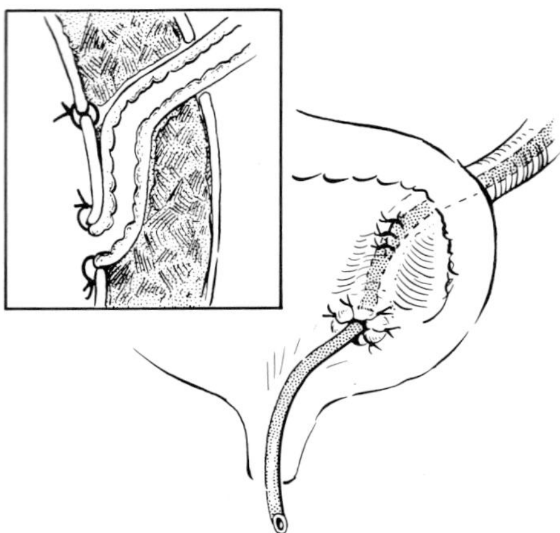

Figure 6.7. Ureteroneocystostomy. The ureter is brought into the bladder following which a submucosal tunnel is created of at least 2 cm length. The ureter is placed beneath the submucosal tunnel, spatulated, and sutured to the bladder wall.

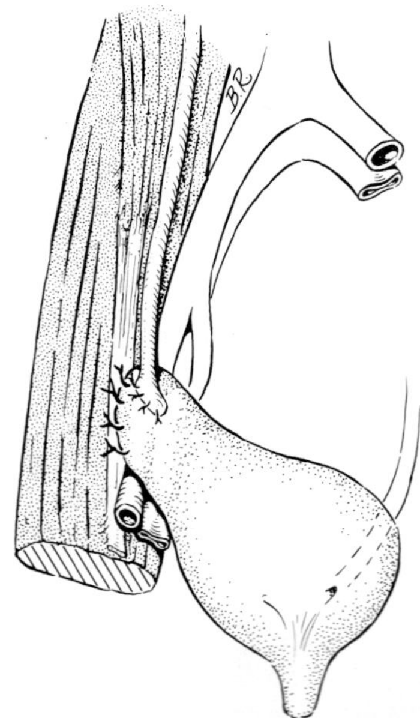

Figure 6.8. Psoas bladder hitch. The bladder is mobilized, during the process of which the contralateral superior vesical artery is ligated and severed. After sufficient mobility is obtained it is sutured to the psoas minor tendon when present or the psoas major muscle.

Hyperchloremic metabolic acidosis may also occur as a complication, particularly in patients in whom the ileal segment is long.

Autotransplantation

An alternative method of treating extensive ureteral injuries is by autotransplantation. Patients with extensive pelvic retroperitoneal fibrosis

   TRAUMATIC INJURIES OF THE GENITOURINARY SYSTEM

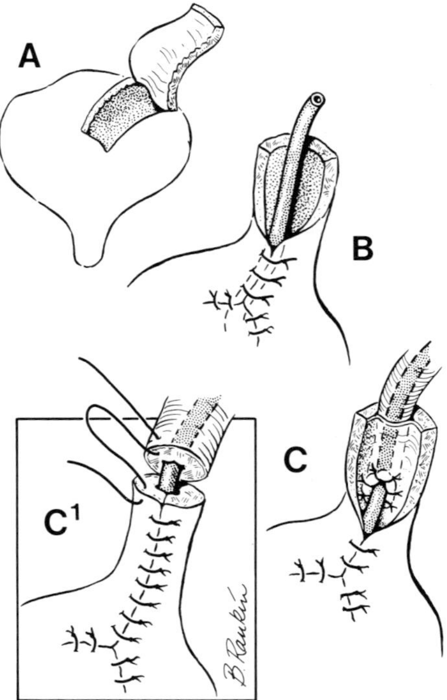

Figure 6.9. Boari pedicle flap. *A*, the pedicle is based on the ipsilateral superior vesical artery and fashioned into a tube (*B*). A psoas hitch is performed and the ureter anastomosed to the end of the tube either end to end (*C'*) or by a submucosal tunnel technique (*C*).

or common and/or internal iliac artery occlusive disease are not candidates for the procedure. The kidney is prepared by mobilizing it and severing the renal artery and vein at their origins. The artery is perfused with cold Ringer's lactate until the venous effluent is clear. The kidney is placed in the previously prepared contralateral iliac fossa and the vessels anastomosed to the common iliac vein and hypogastric artery with 6-0 Prolene. Should the hypogastric artery be inadequate, the renal artery may be anastomosed end-to-side to the common iliac artery. A ureteroneocystostomy completes the procedure. The iliac fossa is drained.

COMPLICATIONS

Numerous complications have been reported following ureteral injuries and include ureteral strictures (Fig. 6.12), fistulae, calculi, hydronephrosis, pyonephrosis, pelvic and retroperitoneal abscesses, and urinary tract infections. Patients who succumb with ureteral injuries usually do so not as a result of the ureteral trauma but rather as a consequence of an associated injury. Intraperitoneal urinary leakage is particularly lethal in patients who have undergone surgery for traumatic injuries to the pancreas, duodenum, and great vessels. The majority of patients with ureteral injuries, however, do well provided the principles described above are observed. The results are somewhat less spectacular in war injuries. Fifty-

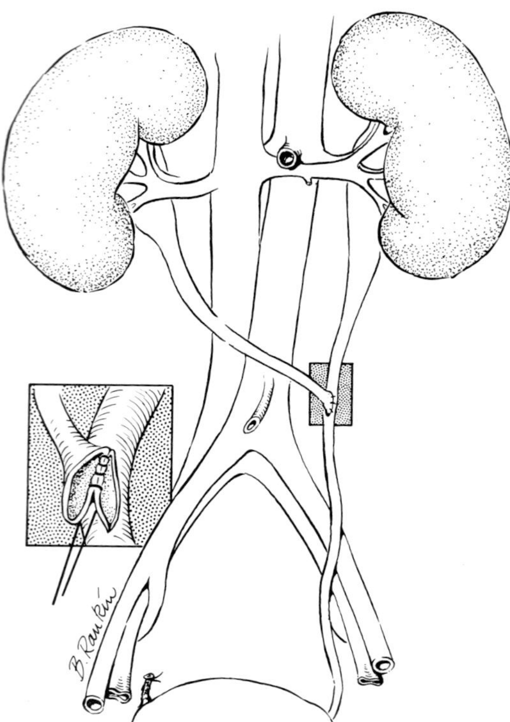

Figure 6.10. Transureteroureterostomy. The injured ureter is brought beneath the mesentery cephalad to the inferior mesenteric artery. The recipient ureter is minimally mobilized and a beveled anastomosis peformed (*insert*).

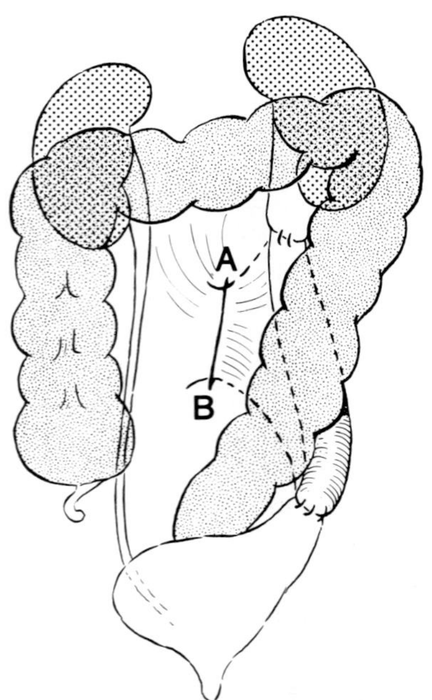

Figure 6.11. Ileal segment substitution. The kidney is completely mobilized and placed caudad. The bladder is mobilized cephalad and a psoas hitch performed. The ileal segment is placed lateral to the colon through a rent in the mesocolon (*A-B*). If a significant segment of viable ureter is present, the proximal anastamosis may be made from bowel to ureter.

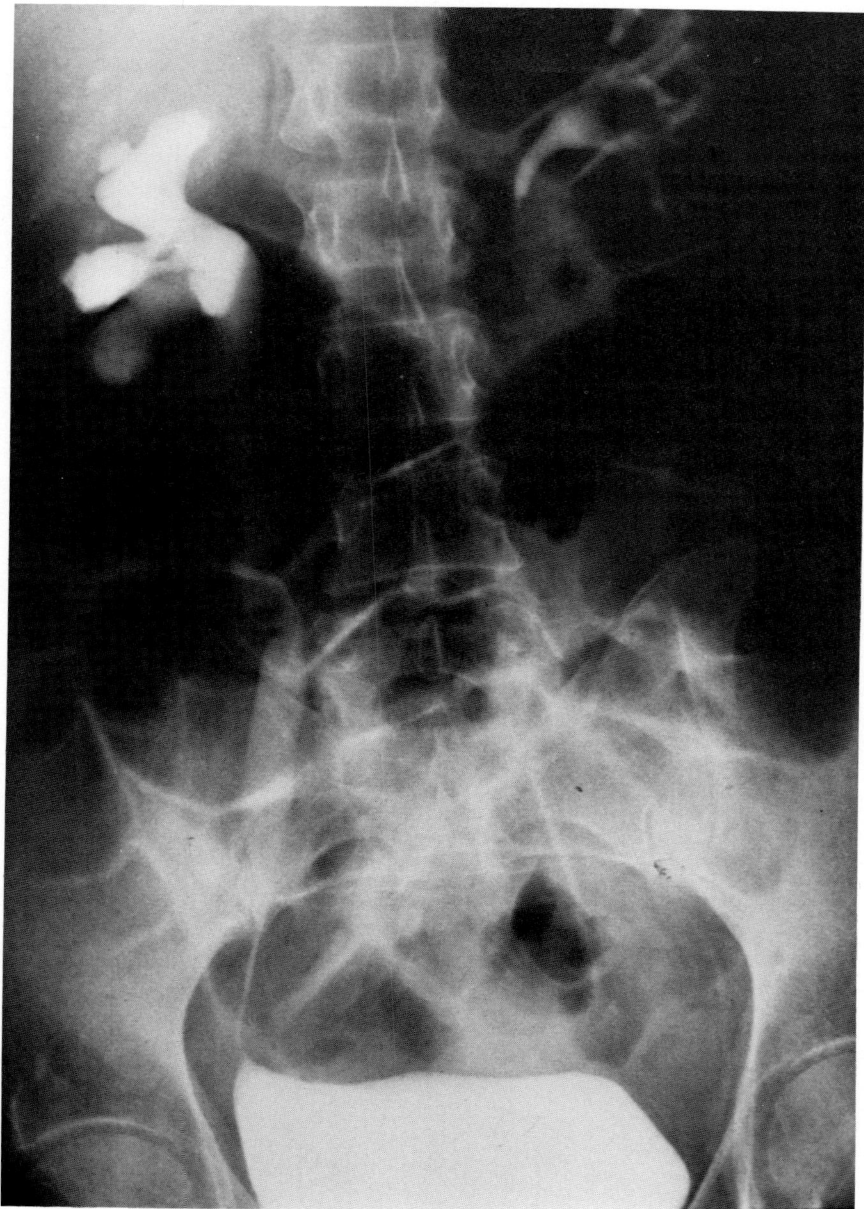

Figure 6.12. Intravenous pyelogram demonstrating a long distal right ureteral stricture which resulted from operative devascularization.

nine percent of ureteral injuries sustained in the Viet Nam conflict had an unsatisfactory outcome.[9]

URETERAL TRAUMA IN CHILDREN

Due to the paucity of retroperitoneal fat in children, blunt trauma accounts for a greater percentage of injuries in the young than it does in the adult; however, in both groups, penetrating injuries account for the vast majority of trauma. Also, ureteropelvic junction disruption resulting from an acute hyperextension injury occurs more frequently in children than adults. Indeed, young boys age five to nine appear to be particularly prone to the injury.[12] The signs, symptoms, diagnosis, and treatment are similar for both adults and children.

REFERENCES

1. Holden, S., Hicks, C. C., O'Brien, D. P., et al. Gunshot wounds of the ureter: a 15-year review of 63 consecutive cases. *J. Urol. 116:*562, 1976.
2. Liroff, S. A., Pontes, J. E. S., and Pierce, J. M., Jr. Gunshot wounds of the ureter: 5 years experience. *J. Urol. 118:*551, 1977.
3. Bright, T. C., and Peters, P. C. Ureteral injuries due to external violence: 10 years experience with 59 cases. *J. Trauma 17:*616, 1977.
4. Carlton, C. E., Jr., Scott, R., Jr., and Guthrie, A. G. The initial management of ureteral injuries: a report of 78 cases. *J. Urol. 105:*335, 1971.
5. Hoch, W. H., Kursh, E. D., and Persky, L. Early, aggressive management of intraoperative ureteral injuries. *J. Urol. 114:*530, 1975.
6. Mendey, R., and McGinty, D. M. The management of delayed recognized ureteral injuries. *J. Urol. 119:*192, 1978.
7. McDougal, W. S., and Persky, L. Nonoperative treatment of ureteral injuries. *J. Urol.,* in press.
8. Walker, J. A. Injuries of the ureter due to external violence. *J. Urol. 102:*410, 1969.
9. Stutzman, R. E. Ballistics and the management of ureteral injuries from high velocity missiles. *J. Urol. 118:*947, 1977.
10. Sieben, D. M., Howerton, L., Amin, M., et al. The role of ureteral stenting in the management of surgical injury of the ureter. *J. Urol. 119:*330, 1978.
11. Raney, A. M. Ureteral trauma: effects of ureteral ligation with and without deligation—experimental studies and case reports. *J. Urol. 119:*326, 1978.
12. Rusche, C., and Morrow, J. W. Injury to the ureter. In *Urology* 3rd ed. Edited by M. F. Campbell and J. H. Harrison. W. B. Saunders Co., Philadelphia, 1970.

7

Renal Injuries

Despite the protection offered by the rib cage, vertebral column, and investing fascia, traumatic injuries of the kidney are not uncommon. Those affected are predominatly males between the ages of 20 and 40 years. The injury is the result of either blunt or penetrating trauma. Blunt trauma in the civilian population accounts for approximately 60% of injuries. The kidney may be injured as a result of a direct blow sustained to the flank or abdomen or as a consequence of an indirect deceleration type injury. In the latter case, the forward momentum of the kidney continues after the body's forward motion is abruptly stopped. Tension on the vascular pedicle results in an intimal tear or frank rupture. Penetrating injuries vary in frequency depending upon the population served but predominate in military conflicts. Both renal units suffer a similar incidence of injury.

Renal trauma is often associated with other injuries. Indeed, 60 to 80% of patients with renal trauma will have concomitant involvement of another organ system.[1] Conversely, 8% of patients with penetrating injuries will have a renal injury.[2] In descending order of occurrence, the most commonly associated traumatic injuries involve the liver, colon, lung, spleen, small bowel, stomach, pancreas, duodenum, and diaphragm.

SIGNS AND SYMPTOMS

Because other injuries are so commonly associated with renal trauma, and because the associated injuries often require emergent therapy, the possibility of a renal injury may not be considered. It is therefore necessary to maintain a high index of suspicion so that significant lesions of the kidney will not be missed. The symptoms are those of localized pain and, on occasion, renal colic when clots or fragments of kidney obstruct the collecting system. The signs of renal injury include hematuria, flank mass, fractured ribs overlying the kidney and ecchymoses or entrance wounds of the lateral abdomen and flank. Hematuria occurs in 80 to 90% of patients with renal trauma[3,4] and, when present, is highly suggestive of injury. However, the absence of hematuria in no way precludes the possibility of a significant renal injury. Indeed, 65% of patients with major renal vascular injuries have clear urine.[1] Although there is a high incidence of hematuria in the first voided specimen postinjury, it is often a fleeting sign since the urine frequently is clear on subsequent voidings.

DIAGNOSIS

Plain Film (KUB)

The plain film of the abdomen is easily obtained and can yield information of great value. Unfortunately, in about 85% of cases, it is unremarkable.[3] Rib fractures overlying the kidney, fractures of the transverse processes or vertebral bodies, obliteration of the psoas shadow or renal outline, a soft tissue mass, displacement of bowel loops, elevation of the diaphragm, scoliosis, and foreign bodies in the region of the kidney are suggestive of renal injury.

Infusion Pyelography with Tomography

The infusion pyelogram is successfully performed when the systolic blood pressure is above 90 mm Hg by infusing 120 cc of radiocontrast over a 5-minute period. When combined with nephrotomography, the pyelogram has a diagnostic accuracy of 95%.[5] The osmotic load presented to the kidney causes a brisk diuresis and, therefore, adequate intravenous fluids must accompany the dye injection. Moreover, the elderly and, in particular, patients who are dehydrated may suffer symptoms of cerebral dehydration from the large osmotic load[6] emphasizing the need for adequate fluid intake prior to, during, and following the study. The roentgenographic findings which suggest renal injury include delayed excretion, decreased concentration of contrast material within the parenchyma, and enlargement of the renal outline. The latter suggests a subcapsular or intrarenal hematoma. Filling defects within the collecting system or nonvisualization of a calyx may be caused by blood clots, renal papallae or an intrarenal hematoma. A radiolucency within the kidney implies a laceration with separation of parenchymal tissue. Finally, the kidney may not visualize suggesting congenital or iatrogenic absence or a pedicle or significant parchenymal injury. The pyelogram is not only helpful in evaluating the injured side but is very useful for determining the integrity, presence, and function of the contralateral renal unit.

Renal Scan

Renal scans have been advocated as a helpful adjunct in diagnosis. They are safe, simple to perform, and result in very little radiation exposure (less than 1 rad). The radioactive material is injected intravenously. Its uptake by the kidney depends upon both the integrity of renal blood flow as well as adequate renal function. It is useful in determining the presence of renal blood flow and significant parchenchymal injury

(Fig. 7.1). It has found its greatest application in following patients postinjury who are treated conservatively rather than as an initial diagnostic modality. Several reports indicate that there is a high degree of correlation between findings observed by scan and those observed by angiography.[7]

Ultrasonography

Sonographic visualization of the kidney is playing an increasingly important role in the management of renal trauma. It is safe, requires little time, and the equipment can be brought to the patient. It is helpful in determining the integrity of the renal parenchyma and locating the position of hematomas: extrarenal, subcapsular, or intrarenal.

Angiography

Patients who should have an angiogram include those who have nonvisualization or decreased visualization of the kidney on intravenous pyelography, individuals in whom extravasation of contrast, persistent hematuria, or continued bleeding occur, and those in whom a pedicle injury is suspected. Findings include no injury, main renal artery occlusion, branch artery occlusion, parenchymal injury, intrarenal hematoma, arteriovenous fistula, and pseudoaneurysm. A hematoma is indicated by displacement of intrarenal and/or capsular vessels or pruning of the small peripheral cortical vessels. Fractures of the parenchyma are suggested by a lucent area within the renal shadow. It is important to note that major branch occlusions are almost always associated with parenchymal tears[8] (Fig. 7.2).

Retrograde Pyelography

Retrograde pyelography is seldom necessary in the evaluation of the renal trauma patient. Moreover, the presence of associated injuries often

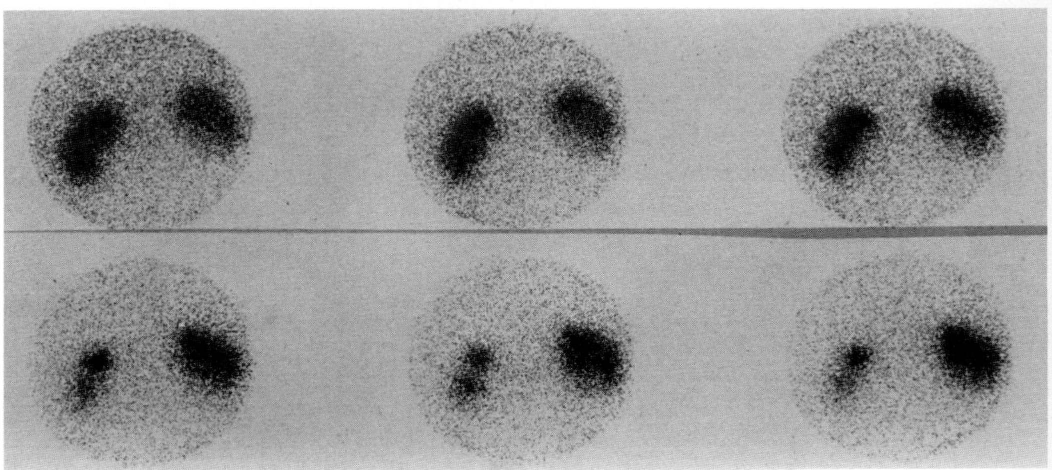

Figure 7.1. Renal scan illustrating a fractured left lower pole. Notice the absence of radioactivity in the region of the lower pole.

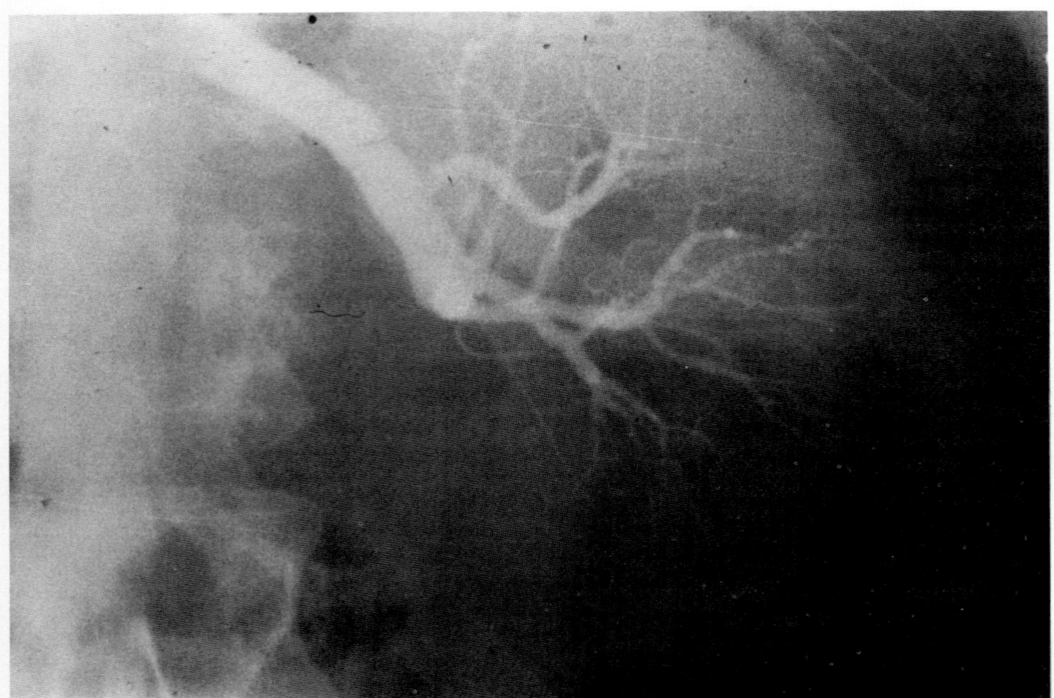

Figure 7.2. Angiogram demonstrating a major arterial branch occlusion associated with a lower pole laceration.

precludes proper positioning, making the procedure difficult and uncomfortable for the patient. Retrograde pyelograms are useful for ruling out obstruction by clots or fragments of kidney when a nonvisualizing renal unit cannot be studied in any other way. They may be helpful when angiography is indicated but cannot be accomplished for technical reasons. It is also used on rare occasions to define the extent of an isolated renal pelvic injury.

CLASSIFICATION OF INJURIES

Renal injuries are classified into one of four groups depending upon the severity of the injury: 1) contusions, 2) lacerations, 3) severe fractures, and 4) pedicle injuries (Fig. 7.3).

Contusions

Renal contusions account for approximately 85% of all kidney injuries. They include subcapsular hematomas and minor cortical lacerations without collecting system involvement. Hematuria is commonly present and may persist, on rare occasions, for a week or more. The plain film rarely is helpful; however, the intravenous pyelogram and nephrotomograms may reveal an irregular or enlarged renal outline. If the intravenous pyelogram is normal and the renal outlines are adequately visualized, no

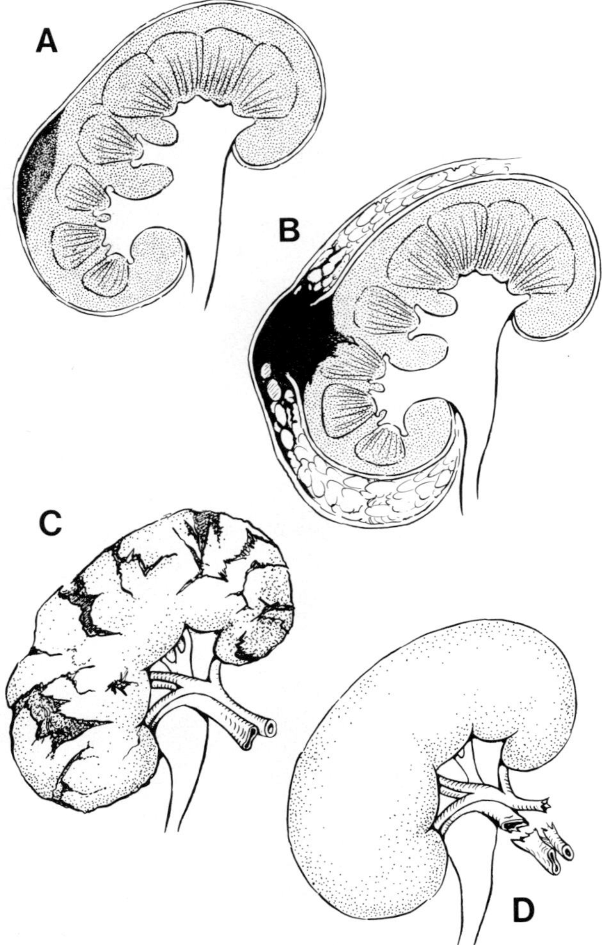

Figure 7.3. Classification of renal trauma. *A*, contusion; *B*, laceration; *C*, severe fracture of the kidney, and *D*, renal pedicle injury.

further diagnostic studies are necessary. Ultrasonography can be helpful in demonstrating the location of the hematoma (Fig. 7.4). Angiographic findings may reveal lack of filling of the small peripheral vessels, and/or displacement of intrarenal or capsular vessels.

Lacerations

Lacerations which extend deep into the parenchyma of the kidney account for less than 10% of all renal trauma. The renal collecting system may or may not be involved. The plain film may reveal a lack of continuity of the renal outline. The intravenous pyelogram may reveal a lucent area within the parenchyma (Fig. 7.5) or extravasation of dye. Sonography confirms the lack of contiguous renal parenchyma. Angiography reveals disrupted peripheral vessels with a wedge-shaped lucent area (Fig. 7.6).

RENAL INJURIES   115

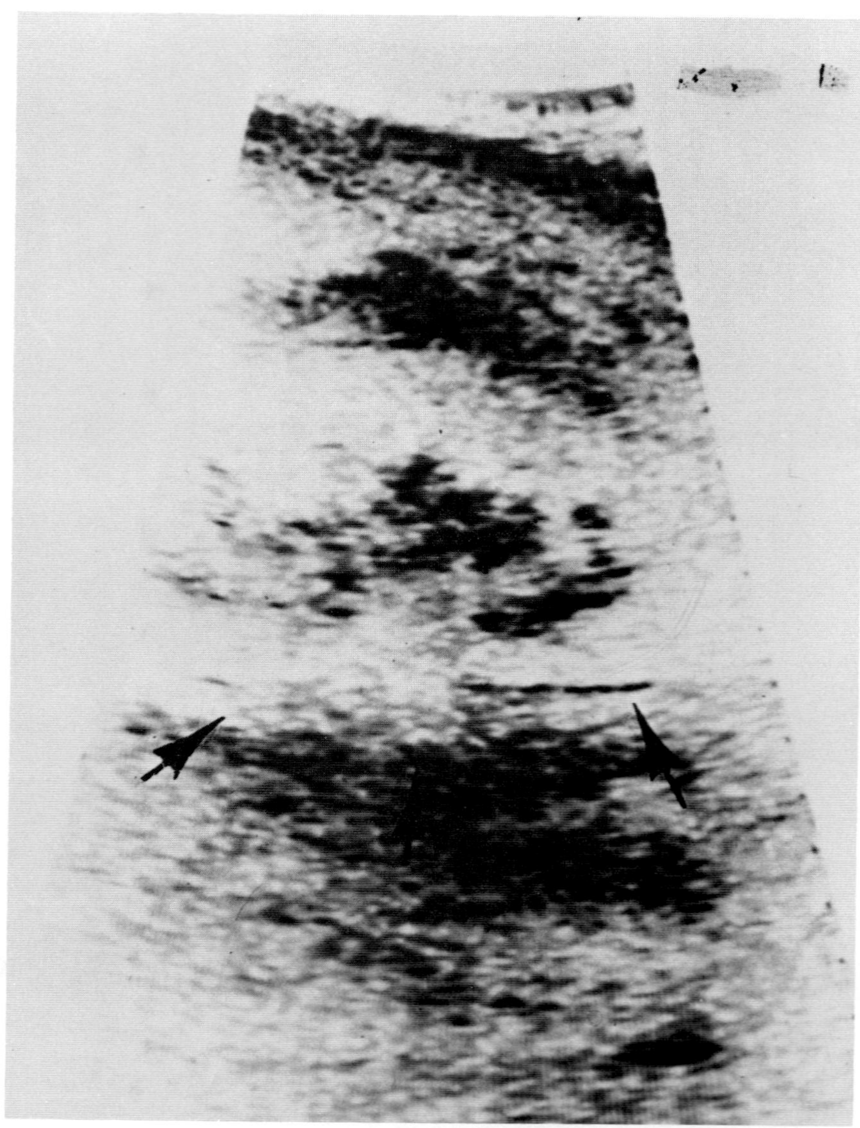

Figure 7.4. Ultrasonogram of a contusion of the kidney demonstrating a subcapsular hematoma (*arrows* point to the hematoma).

Severe Fractures

Severe fractures involve deep lacerations of multiple portions of renal parenchyma. The collecting system is invariably disrupted. The injury has, on occasion, been referred to as a pulped kidney. The intravenous pyelogram usually reveals delayed or no visualization. Extravasation of dye, absence of a continuous renal outline, and fragmented portions of kidney may also be observed. Angiography may reveal main renal artery or branch artery occlusions, extravasation, or fragmentation of the parenchyma (Fig. 7.7).

     TRAUMATIC INJURIES OF THE GENITOURINARY SYSTEM

Pedicle Injuries

Vascular injuries of the renal pedicle include lacerations or disruptions of the vessels and tears of the arterial intima. The latter is usually the result of a deceleration type injury. The tear occurs within 1 cm of the junction of the renal artery with the aorta. Intimal tears generally lead to thrombosis of the entire vessel (Fig. 7.8). The majority of patients have an unstable blood pressure or a palpable flank mass and significant associated injuries. Sixty-five percent of patients do not have hematuria.[1] Intravenous pyelography reveals nonvisualization of the affected side. Angiography demonstrates the lesion.

TREATMENT

Contusions

Renal contusions are treated nonoperatively with bed rest and serial monitoring of vital signs and hematocrit. If hematuria is initially present, it frequently clears within several days; however, rarely it may persist for a week or more. These patients generally do well and complications are few (vide infra).

Lacerations

The treatment of patients with major lacerations of the renal parenchyma, with or without collecting system involvement, is controversial.

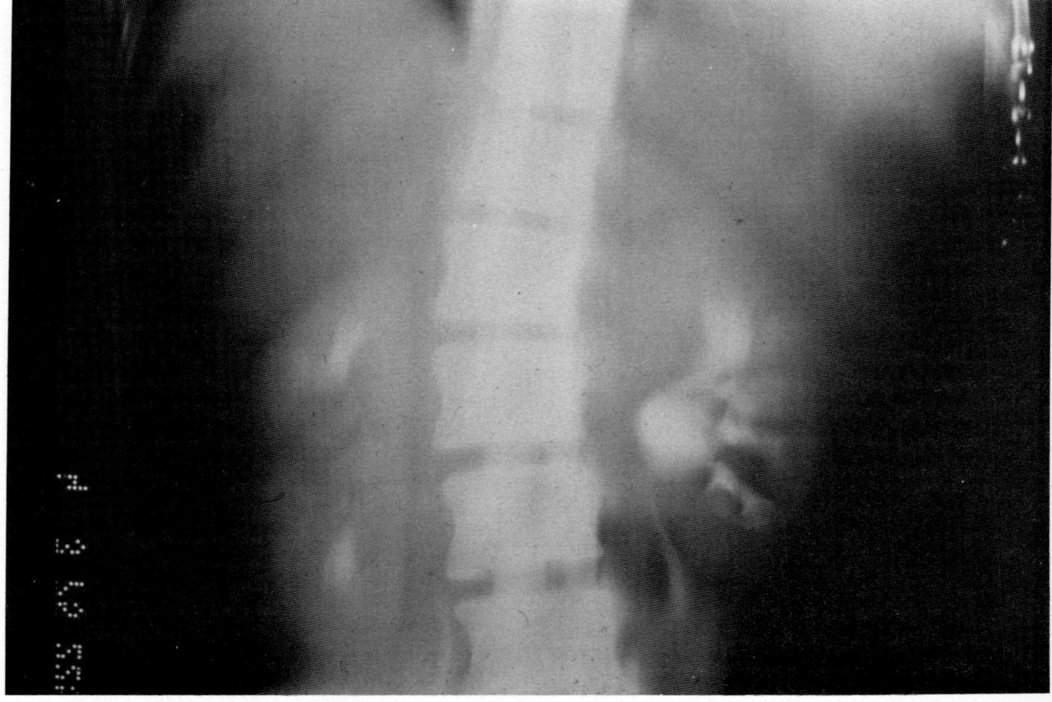

Figure 7.5. Nephrotomogram illustrating a laceration of the right kidney.

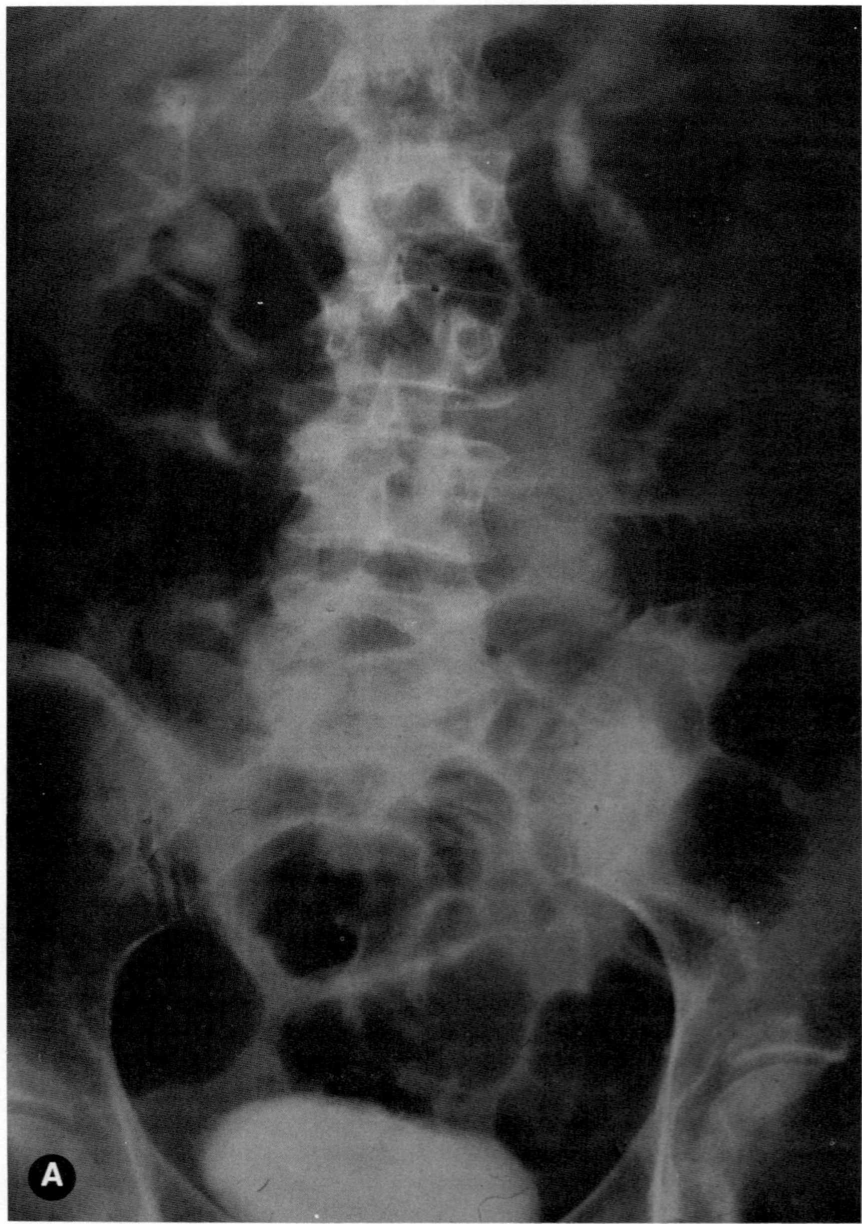

Figure 7.6A. Deep laceration of the kidney. IVP reveals incomplete filling of the calyceal system on the left with extravasation of dye.

The conservative approach, initially advocated by Sargent and Marquardt[9] and McCague,[10] involves careful observation with frequent monitoring of blood pressure and hematocrit and administration of prophylactic antibiotics. Patients are operated upon if they have an expanding flank mass, increasing pain, persistent fever, or bleeding. Using this approach, 4 to 16% of patients require nephrectomy in the postinjury

     TRAUMATIC INJURIES OF THE GENITOURINARY SYSTEM

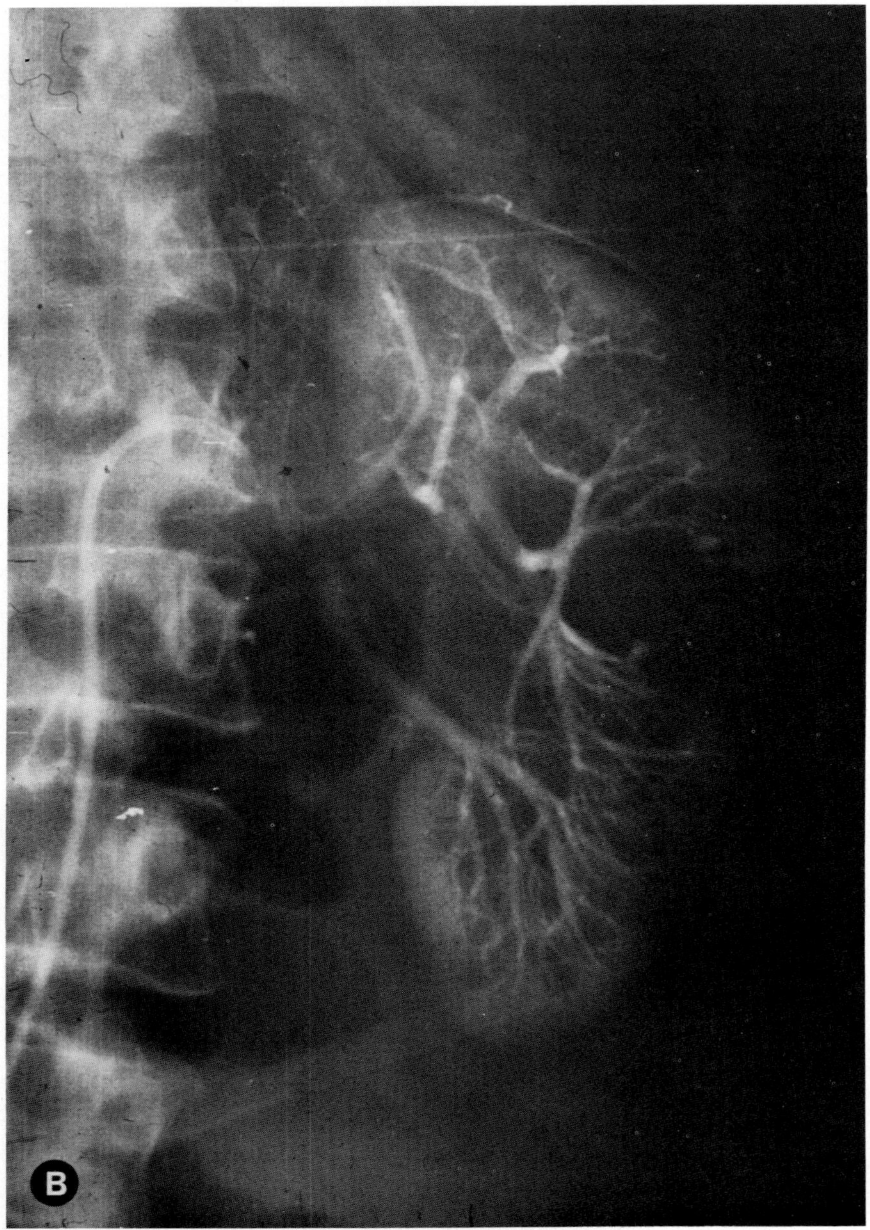

Figure 7.6B. Angiogram demonstrates a mid renal fracture.

period and the complication rate (vide infra) is about 5%.[3, 11-13] Another form of therapy involves immediate exploration and repair of the injury. The proponents of this form of therapy suggest that nonoperative management results in a much higher incidence of complications than noted above and that immediate surgery results in less morbidity. If immediate surgery is undertaken, it is critical that control of the renal pedicle be

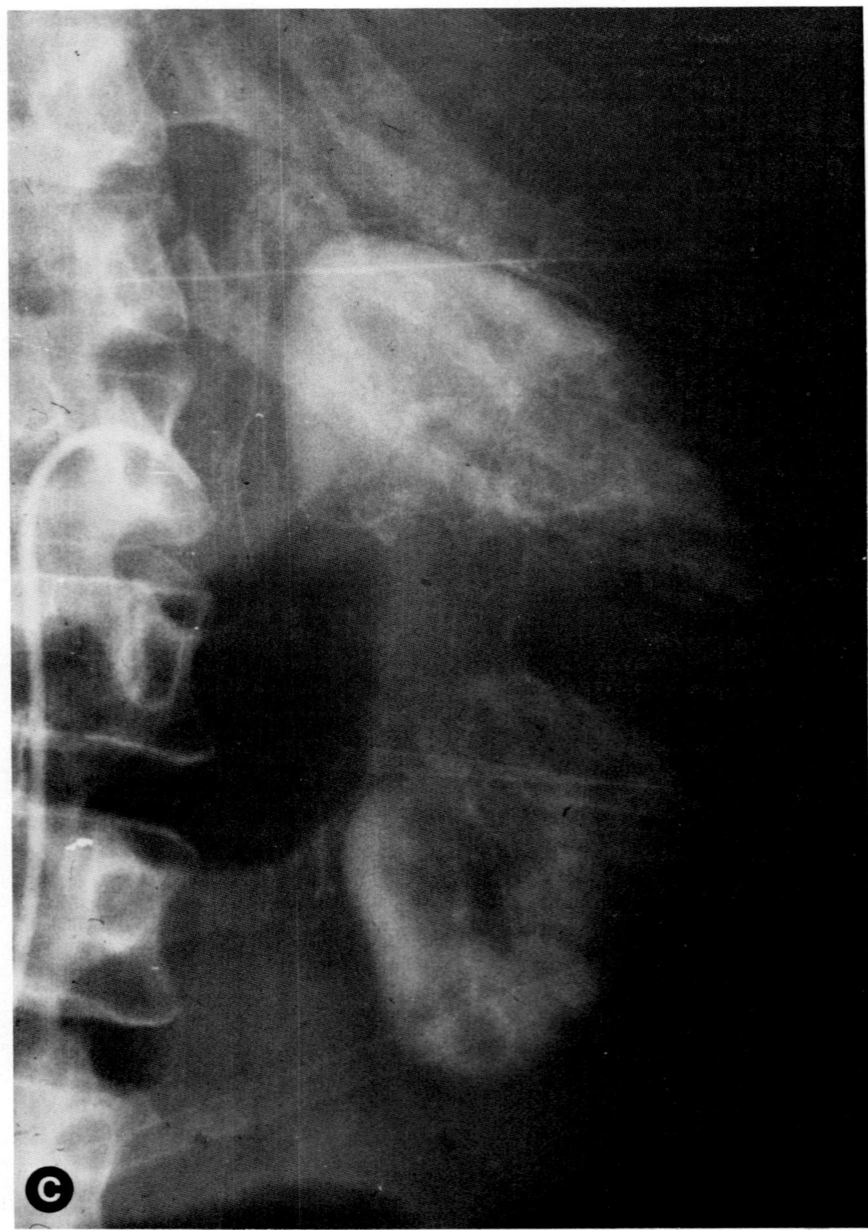

Figure 7.6C.   The nephrogram phase also illustrates the fracture.

gained before Gerota's fascia is entered. Fifty percent of patients explored immediately postinjury who did not have the renal pedicle controlled prior to the incision of Gerota's fascia underwent nephrectomy, whereas there was only a 30% incidence of nephrectomy in those in whom vascular control was obtained initially.[14]

Our experience has led us to employ the conservative approach with

   TRAUMATIC INJURIES OF THE GENITOURINARY SYSTEM

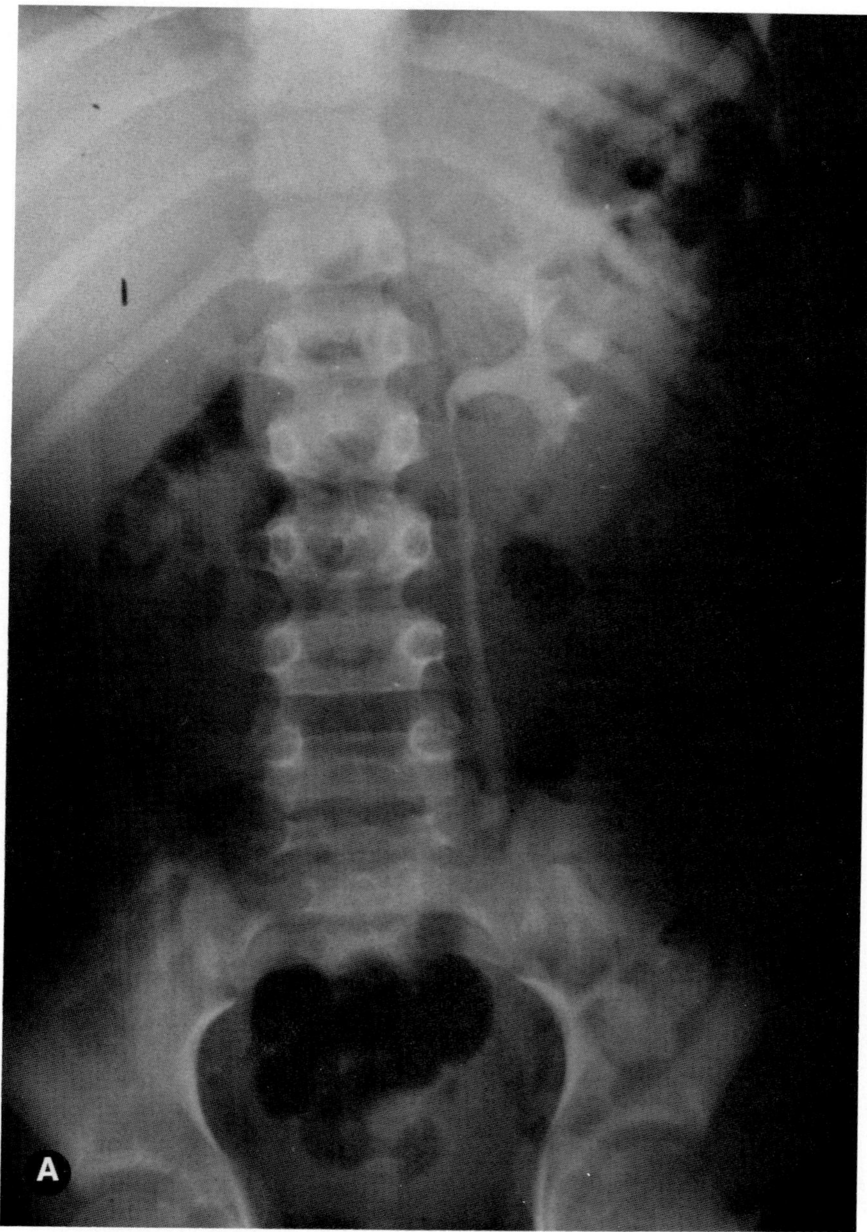

Figure 7.7A. Severe fracture of the kidney. The IVP demonstrates a lack of visualization on the right.

this type of injury unless it is due to penetrating trauma. Penetrating injuries are explored immediately, both because of the high incidence of multiple organ system involvement and because untreated penetrating injuries of the kidney result in a high incidence of complications. Those managed conservatively are monitored as described above and restudied with pyelography, ultrasonography and, when indicated, angiography in

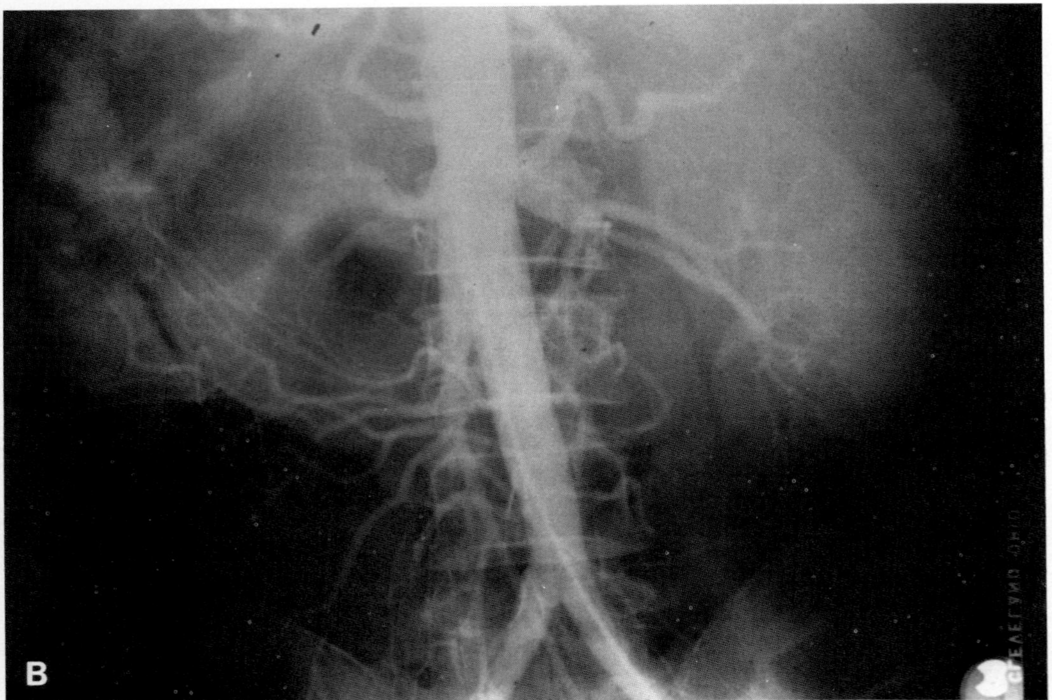

Figure 7.7*B.*   Angiography reveals a complete occlusion of the main renal artery.

the post-traumatic period. When re-evaluated in this manner, those who require surgery are identified and explored within 2 to 5 days postinjury. Using this approach, the complication rate is minimized and maximal preservation of renal tissue is achieved.

Severe Fractures

Severe fractures require immediate exploration after patient stabilization. Antibiotics are administered and the injury approached through the abdomen. Control of the renal pedicle must be obtained prior to opening Gerota's fascia and exposing the kidney. Every attempt is made to preserve as much parenchyma as possible and to achieve a water tight closure of the collecting system. The retroperitoneal space is drained separately and away from other injured retroperitoneal structures, *i.e.* duodenum and pancreas. If this is not accomplished, pancreatic and duodenal fistulae and pyonephrosis are common sequellae.

Pedicle Injuries

Renal pedicle injuries also require immediate exploration. Unfortunately, patients who sustain vascular injuries of the renal pedicle often have multiple renal parechymal lacerations as well, making salvage of the renal unit difficult. Preservation of kidneys with pedicle injuries is more likely to be successful when the injury has not resulted in multiple parenchymal lacerations. Success has been reported with revascularization

    TRAUMATIC INJURIES OF THE GENITOURINARY SYSTEM

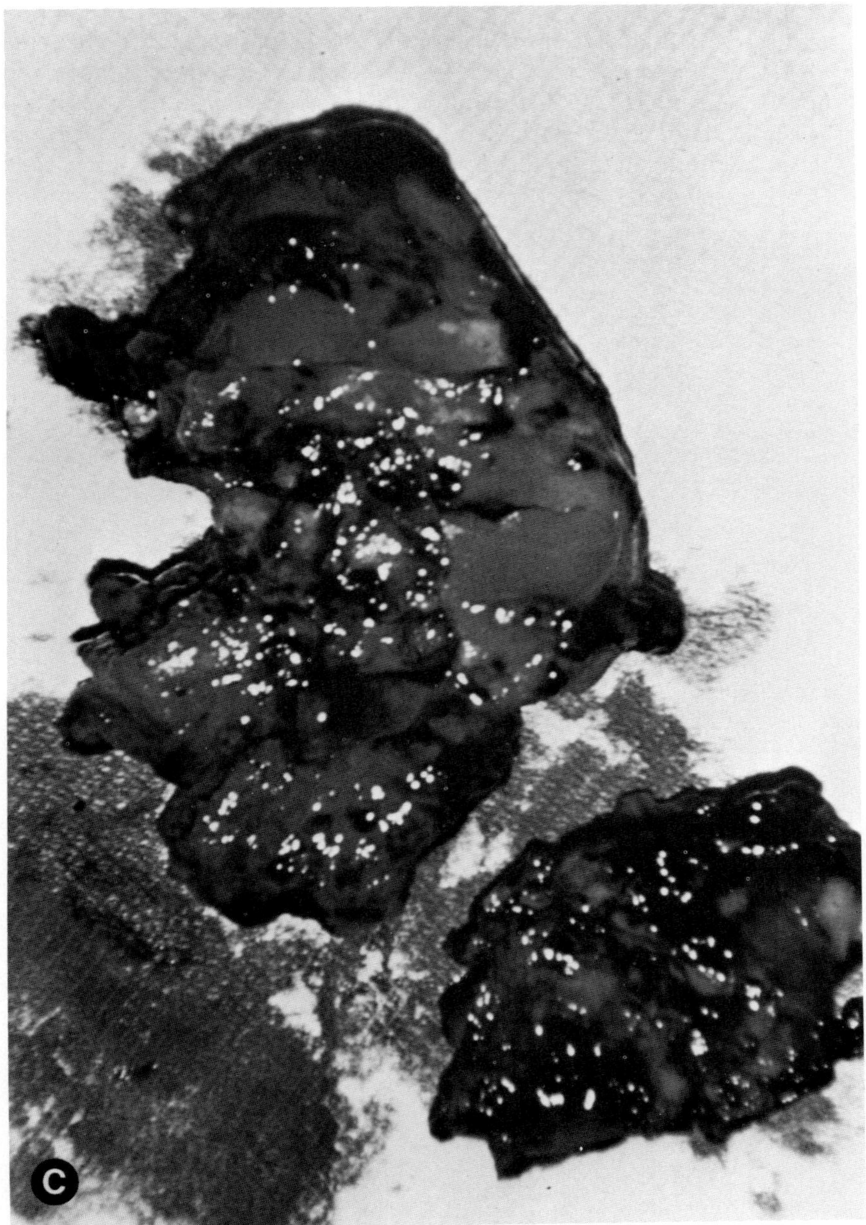

Figure 7.7C. Operative specimen demonstrates the extensive fragmentation of the kidney.

up to 16 hours postinjury,[15] however, the experience of most centers in preserving renal function following pedicle injury is discouraging.

SURGICAL TECHNIQUE

Patients requiring immediate surgical exploration for renal trauma are those who have an expanding flank mass, sustain penetrating injuries,

persist in bleeding, have pedicle injuries, or sustain severe fractures of the
renal unit. Surgery is indicated later in the patient's course for those who
develop infection, have an expanding flank mass, demonstrate a continued
fall in hematocrit, develop renal hypertension, or radiologic evidence of
renal deterioration, or in those whose injuries were not fully appreciated

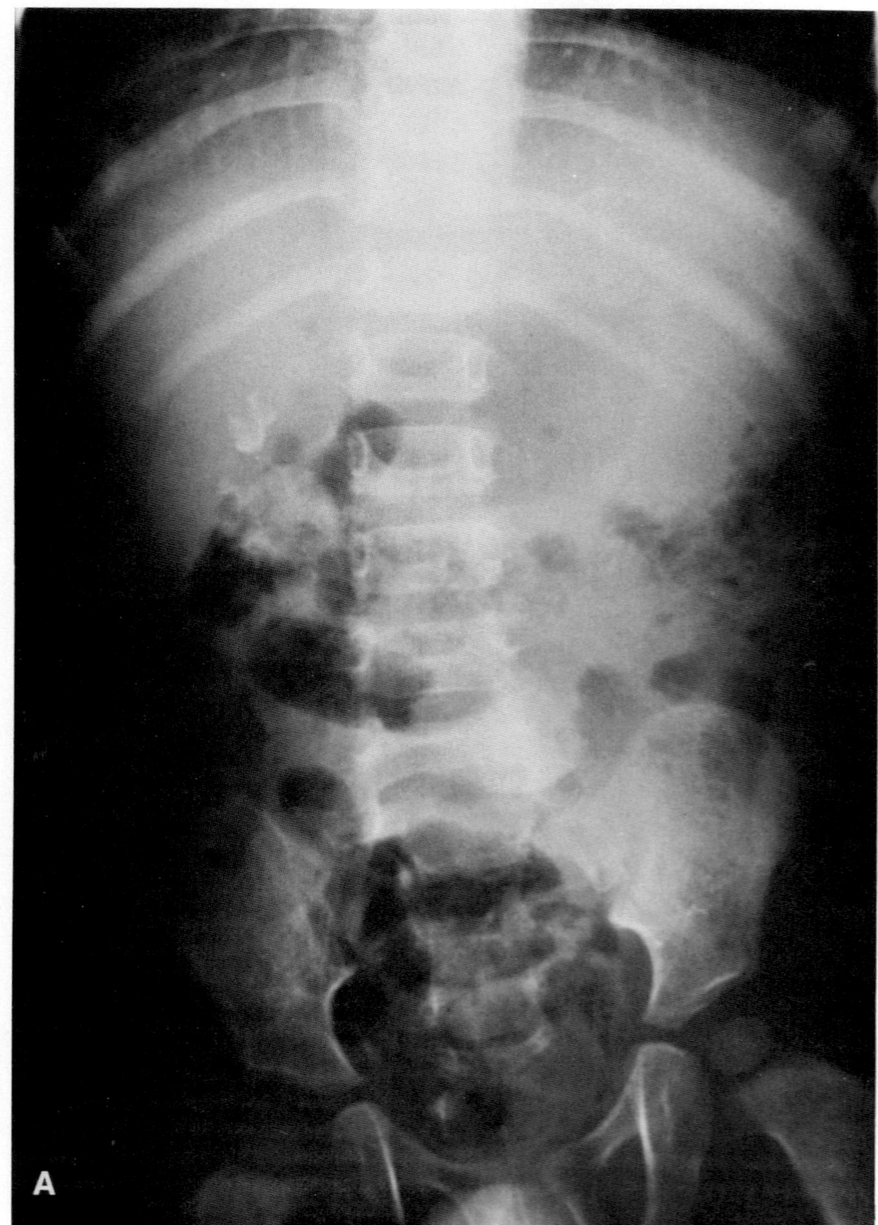

Figure 7.8A. Intimal tear of the left main renal artery. The IVP reveals nonvisualization of the left kidney.

 TRAUMATIC INJURIES OF THE GENITOURINARY SYSTEM

at the time of initial injury. The surgery is ideally performed between the second and fifth day after injury. This allows the patient's general condition to stabilize, and all diagnostic studies to be completed. Surgery at this time permits the conservation of maximal amounts of renal parenchyma. Beyond 5 to 7 days fibrosis and the risk of infection increase considerably.

Patients who are operated upon in the immediate postinjury period are explored through a midline abdominal wound. The status of the contralateral kidney must be known before any manipulation of the injured kidney is performed. If a pyelogram was not obtained preoperatively, intravenous injection of radiocontrast and an intra-operative roentgenogram should be obtained. This, coupled with palpation of the uninjured kidney and its vascular supply to confirm adequate perfusion, will provide the information necessary for proper evaluation of the contralateral renal

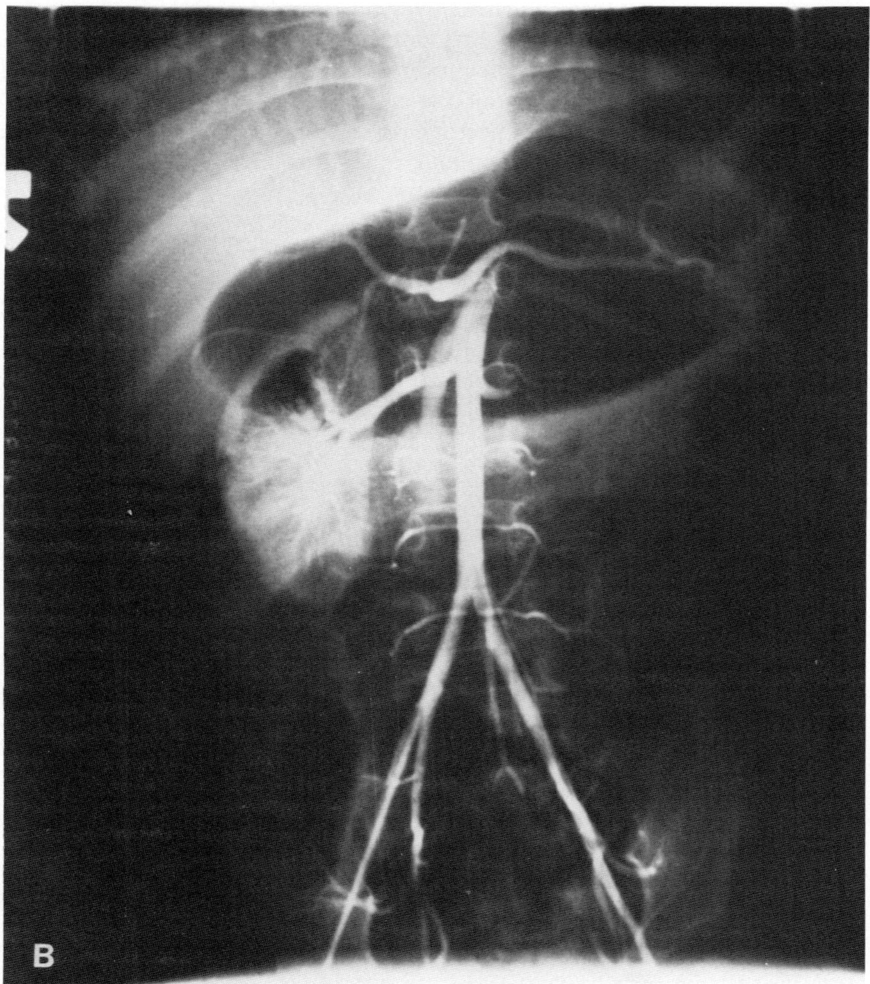

Figure 7.8B. Angiography shows occlusion of the left renal artery.

unit. The renal pedicle of the injured kidney is secured by incising the posterior peritoneum over the aorta at the route of the mesentary (Fig. 7.9). The left renal vein is identified as it crosses over the aorta. By retracting it gently cephalad, the right and left renal arteries can be identified and the appropriate artery encircled with a vascular loop. The renal vein is identified and likewise encircled with a vascular loop. If a significant retroperitoneal hematoma is present, the vasculature may be difficult to identify. Gerota's fascia is opened and the kidney mobilized. If bleeding is brisk, the renal vasculature is occluded with a noncrushing vascular clamp.

If there is obvious destruction of tissue, those fragments of kidney completely separated from the renal parenchyma are removed. Debridement is carried out on those other areas badly damaged. Interlobar and interlobular arteries are controlled with 4-0 or 5-0 atraumatic catgut sutures. If there are large gaps in the parenchyma, they are sutured with vertical mattress sutures and tied over buffers of fat obtained from the perinephric envelope (Fig. 7.10). Occasionally, a large defect may be covered by omentum, peritoneum, or even muscle. In selected cases, a partial nephrectomy is performed (Fig. 7.11). This allows for control of hemorrhage, debridement of necrotic tissue, and salvage of the renal unit. If bleeding seems to be intraluminal, a nephrostomy is indicated. A gap

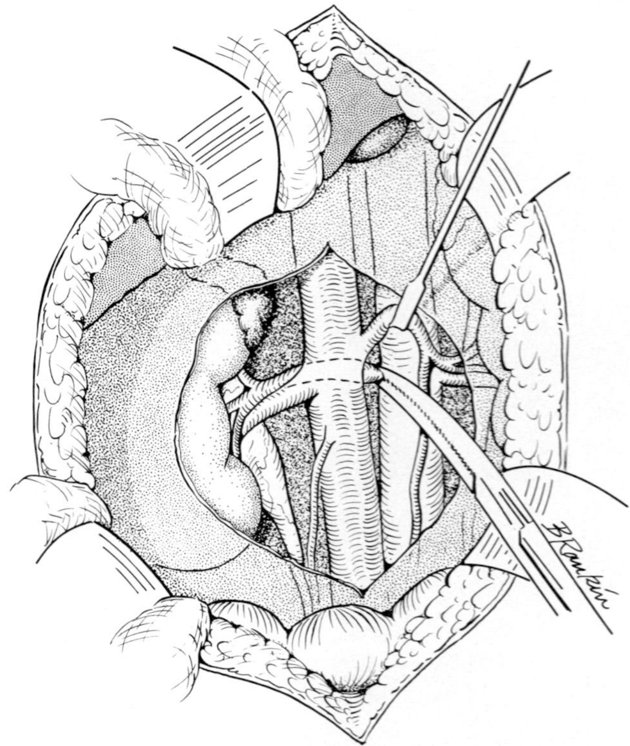

Figure 7.9. Anatomy of the retroperitoneum and renal vasculature. By incising the peritoneum immediately overlying the aorta at the route of the mesentary, the renal vessels are exposed.

   TRAUMATIC INJURIES OF THE GENITOURINARY SYSTEM

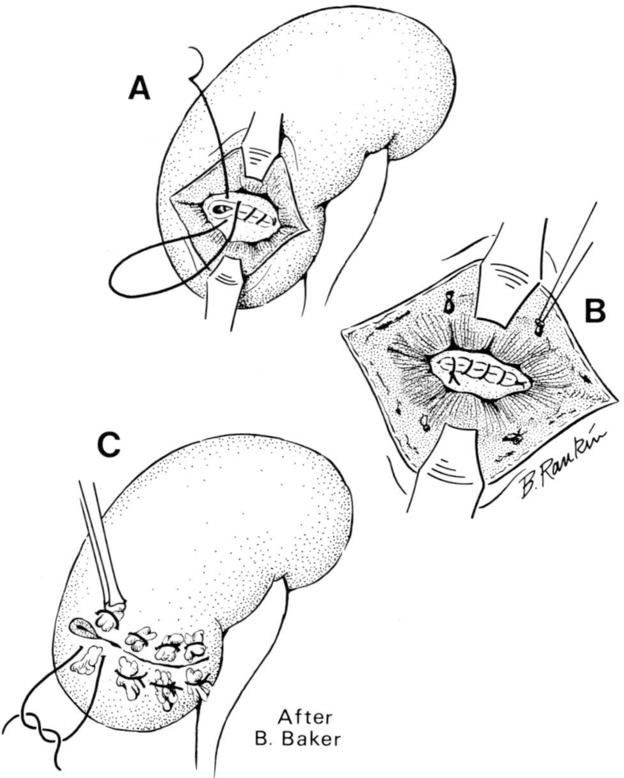

Figure 7.10. *A,* deep lacerations may involve the renal collecting system. *B,* the necrotic tissue is debrided and the collecting system closed in a water tight fashion with fine chromic suture. *C,* hemostasis is achieved by suture ligatures and the capsule and parenchyma reapproximated by mattress sutures placed over buffers of fat.

in the capsule may be covered by a free graft of peritoneum. After debridement is complete and hemorrhage is controlled, the abdomen is carefully inspected for other injuries, a retroperitoneal drain secured, and the abdomen closed. On occasion, the kidney may be severely lacerated; yet, the indeterminate or poor function of the contralateral kidney requires the preservation of the function of the injured kidney. In such circumstances, the hilar vessels are separated close to their insertion from the great vessels. The kidney is placed on the abdominal wall, perfused with cold Ringer's lactate until the venous effluent is clear and placed in slush. After the repair is complete, the kidney is placed in the contralateral iliac fossa. The vessels are anastomosed to the hypogastric artery and iliac vein, and a ureteroneocystostomy performed. It may be possible to do the surgery without severing the ureter, in which case the need for a ureteral anastomosis is obviated.

Pedicle injuries require early control of the vessels as described above. Lacerations of the main renal vein are repaired with a running 6-0 Prolene suture. Branch veins may be ligated since the venous return from the kidney intercommunicates. All renal arterial injuries should be repaired

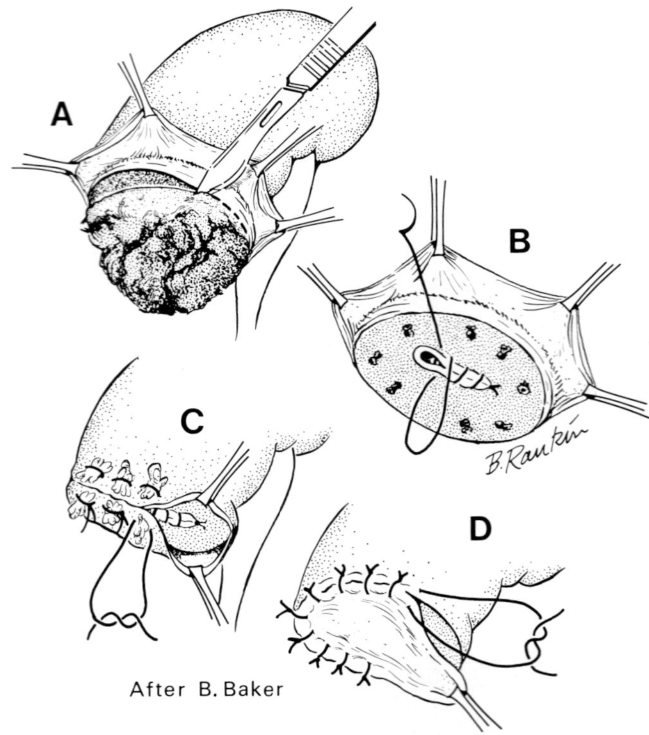

Figure 7.11. Technique of heminephrectomy. *A,* the capsule is dissected free and the necrotic renal parenchyma excised. *B,* blood vessels are individually suture ligated and the collecting system closed with fine chromic suture. *C,* buffers of fat cushion the mattress sutures and the end is covered with capsule or *D,* a free peritoneal graft.

if parenchyma supplied by the vessel is to be retained. Intimal tears may be sutured or the segment with the tear resected and an end-to-end anastomosis performed with 6-0 Prolene (Fig. 7.11). The latter method is generally preferred. Saphenous vein, patch grafts of endogenous or prosthetic material, and prosthetic vascular grafts are used when indicated (Fig. 7.12).

COMPLICATIONS OF RENAL TRAUMA

Complications may be classified as either early or late in occurrence and are generally related to either extravasation or vascular disruption. Early complications or those which occur within the first 6 weeks postinjury include ileus, rebleeding, perinephric abscess, progressive loss of renal function, sepsis, and fistula formation (Figs. 7.13 and 7.14). These complications can be minimized by accurately determining the extent of the injury initially and carefully evaluating the status of the kidney in the first week postinjury. Often times the complications occur as a result of failure to operate in the 2- to 5-day critical period. Late complications include hypertension, hydronephrosis, chronic pyelonephritis, calculus

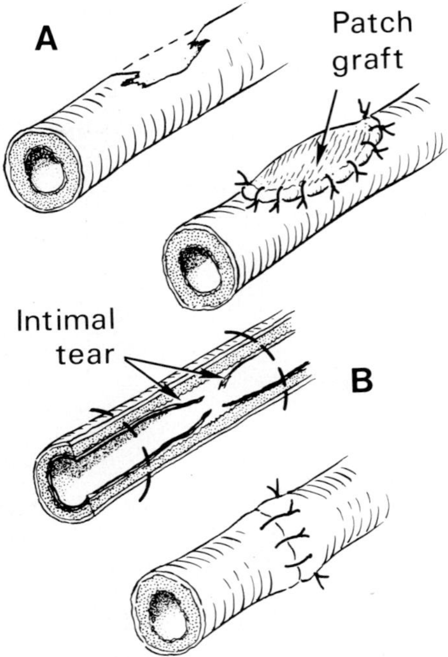

Figure 7.12. Vessels are repaired by an end-to-end anastomosis, by bypass grafts or by the use of patch grafts. *A*, closure of the injured artery with suture will result in a compromised lumen. A patch graft of saphenous vein or prosthetic material allows closure of the defect without compromise of the lumen. This technique reduces the chances of renal artery stenosis and its sequellae in the postoperative period. *B*, intimal tears often result in thrombosis of the vessel. They are often best repaired by resection and end-to-end anastomosis.

formation, arteriovenous fistulae, pseudocyst formation, renal atrophy, capsular hydrocele, and renal artery stenosis. Hypertension is usually the result of perirenal fibrosis with constriction of the parenchyma (Page kidney, Fig. 7.15), or renal artery branch occlusions. The elevated blood pressure is mediated by the renin-angiotensin system. Arteriovenous fistulae may also result in hypertension (Fig. 7.16). The treatment of choice is complete removal of the diseased area since results with more conservative operative approaches, especially for correction of hypertension secondary to arteriovenous fistulae[16] have met with failure. All trauma patients should have an intravenous pyelogram before discharge and at 6 months postinjury. This allows for early detection of impending complications.

RENAL INJURY IN CHILDREN

Children are more vulnerable to renal injury than are adults. The retroperitoneal area is not as well protected and the relative size of the kidney is greater in the child than in the adult. Blunt trauma accounts for the majority of injuries and males predominate, although not to the extent

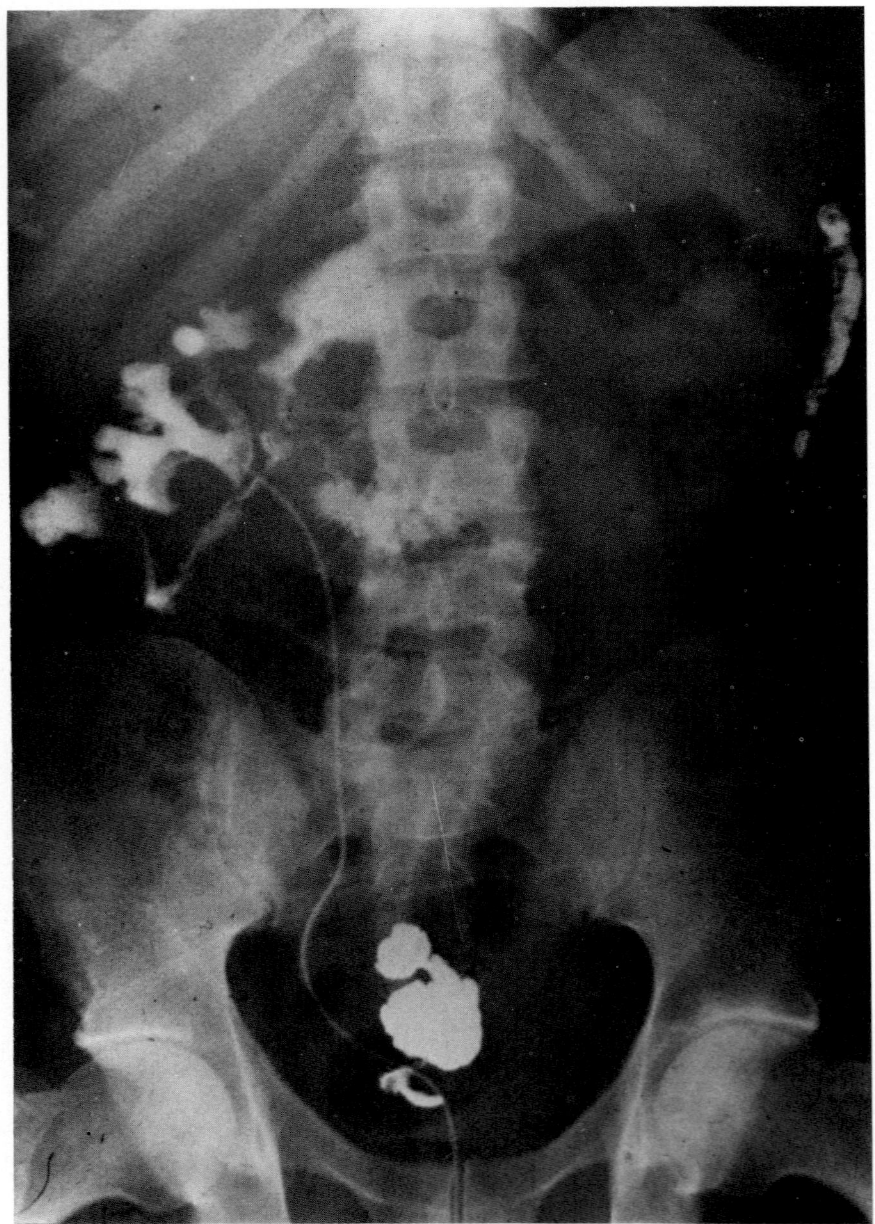

Figure 7.13. Pyeloduodenal fistula. Retrograde pyelogram in a patient who sustained a gun shot wound 3 months previously. Notice the dye in the duodenum.

they do in the adult population.[17] One-fifth of children with renal injury have been found to have pre-existing renal disease.[18] These diseases include hydronephrosis, ecotpia, tumor, megaureter, and hypoplasia (Fig. 7.17). Even a low degree of impact may produce hematuria, and careful evaluation is required to discover the underlying disease. In our experi-

     TRAUMATIC INJURIES OF THE GENITOURINARY SYSTEM

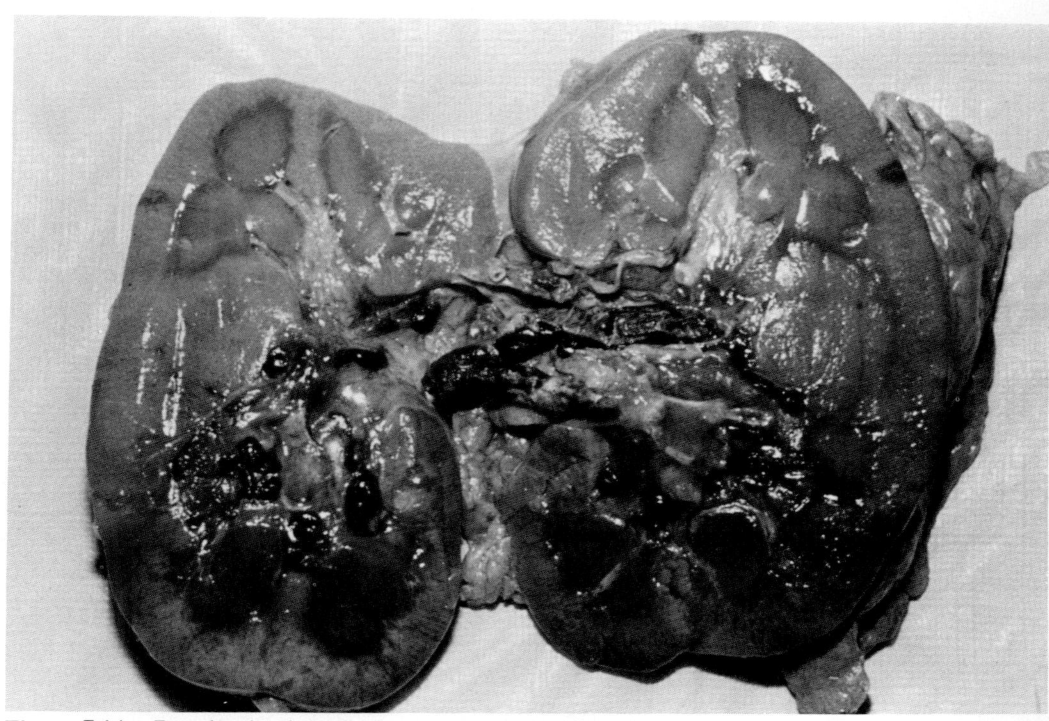

Figure 7.14. Renal vein thrombosis following a traumatic blow to the flank. Notice the complete occlusion of the main branch of the renal vein.

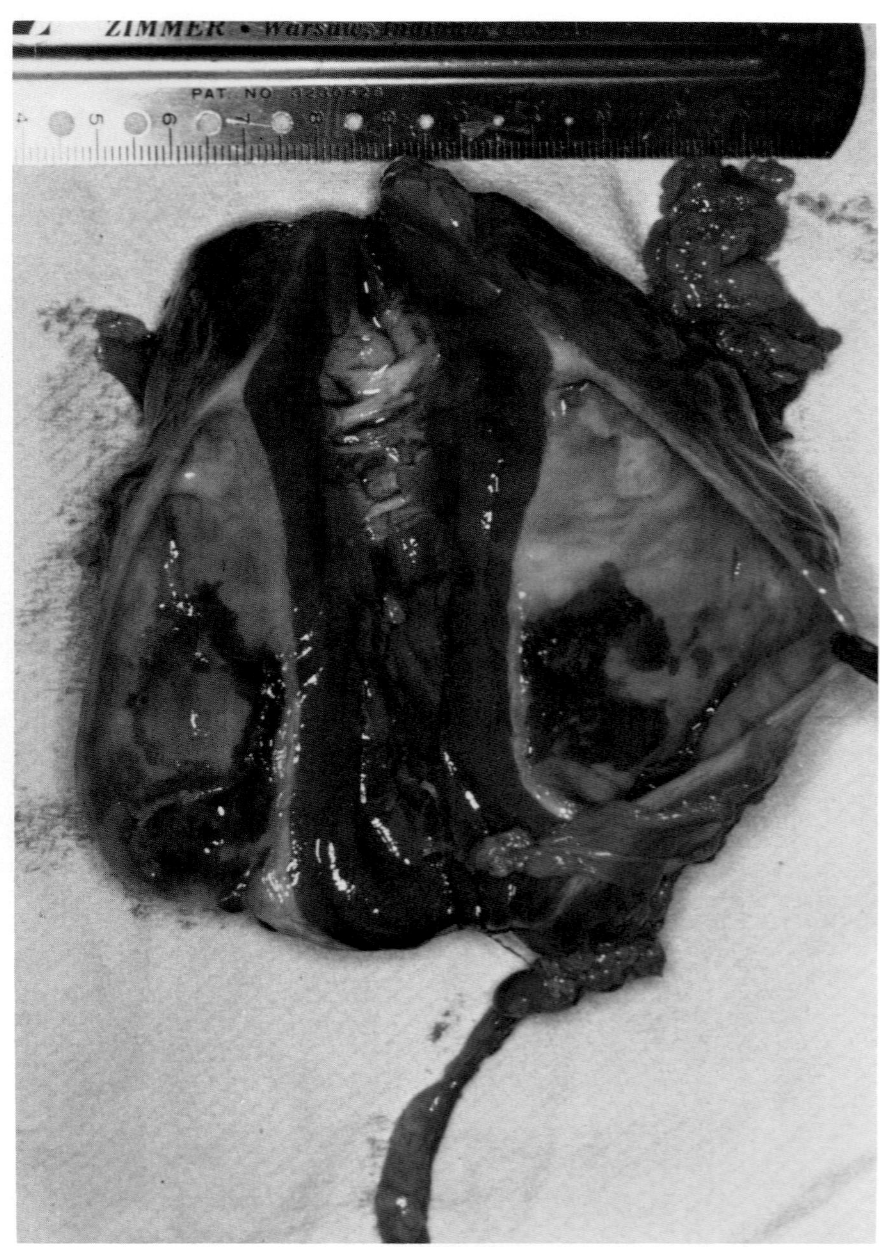

Figure 7.15. Page kidney. Postinjury the patient developed hypertension. The operative specimen demonstrates compression of the renal parenchyma by perirenal fibrosis.

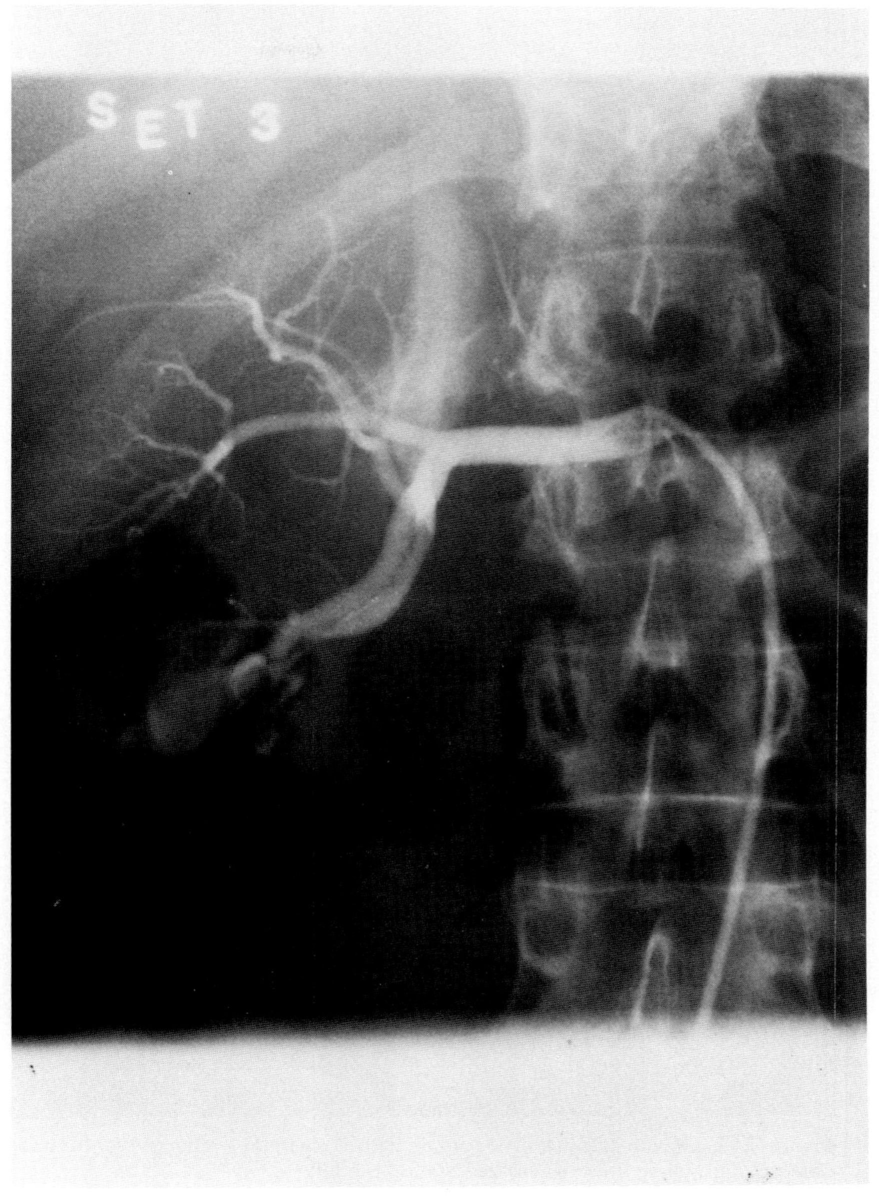

Figure 7.16. An arteriovenous fistula demonstrated by angiography in a patient who sustained a stab wound to the flank a year previously.

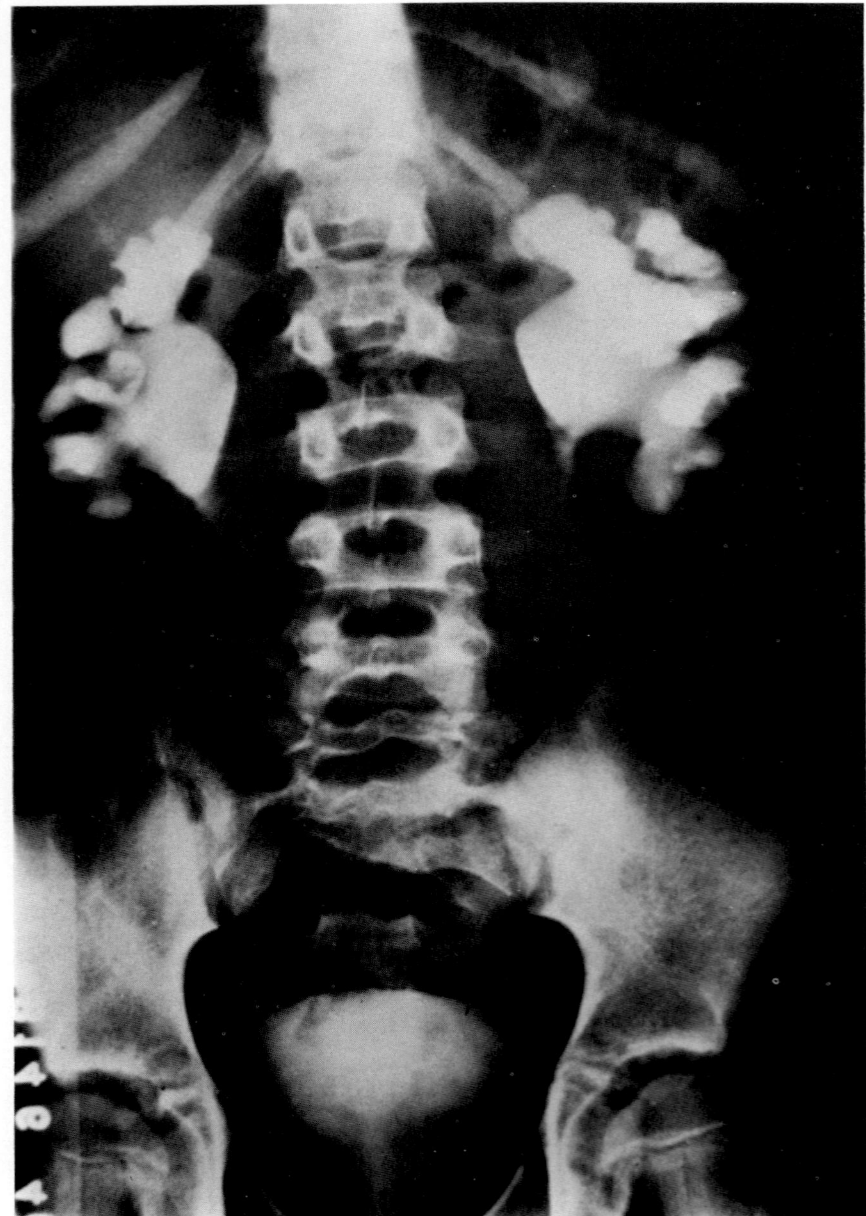

Figure 7.17. Renal trauma in a patient with congenital ureteropelvic junction obstruction. Notice the extravasated dye on the left.

ence, the incidence of contusion, laceration, severe fractures, and pedicle injuries are comparable to adults.[19] Conservation of renal parenchyma is of prime importance in the young and every attempt is made to salvage all viable tissue. The patient is stabilized and those who require surgery are operated at 2 to 5 days postinjury when possible. This results in a lesser incidence of nephrectomy and an increased degree of renal paren-

     TRAUMATIC INJURIES OF THE GENITOURINARY SYSTEM

chyma preservation. A delay of more than 5 days increases the incidence of urinoma formation, fibrosis, fistulae, and infection. Of course, children with pedicle injuries, penetrating trauma, and expanding flank masses require immediate surgery.

REFERENCES

1. Hai, M. A., Pontes, J. E., and Pierce, J. M., Jr. Surgical management of major renal trauma: a review of 102 cases treated by conservative surgery. *J. Urol. 118*:7, 1977.
2. Tynberg, P., Hoch, W. H., Persky, L., et al. The management of renal injuries coincident with penetrating wound of the abdomen. *J. Trauma 13*:502, 1973.
3. Glenn, J. F., and Harvard, B. M. The injured kidney. *J.A.M.A. 173*:1189, 1960
4. Banowsky, L. H., Wolfel, D. A., and Lackner, L. H. Considerations in diagnosis and management of renal trauma. *J. Trauma 10*:587, 1970.
5. Mahoney, S. A., and Persky, L. Intravenous drip nephrotomography as an adjunct in the evaluation of renal injury. *J. Urol. 99*:513, 1968.
6. Rieser, C. Diagnostic evaluation of suspected genito-urinary tract injury. *J.A.M.A. 199*: 714, 1967.
7. Freeman, L. M., Kay, D. J., and Meng, C. H. The contribution of renal scanning in the evaluation of renal trauma. *Radiology 86*:102, 1966.
8. Moss, D. I., and Freeman, R. Renal angiography and the management of severe closed renal trauma. *Aust. N.Z. J. Surg. 47*:462, 1977.
9. Sargent, J. C., and Marquardt, C. R. Renal injuries. *J. Urol. 63:*1, 1950.
10. McCague, E. J. Renal trauma: conservative management. *J. Urol. 63:*773, 1950.
11. Morrow, J. W., and Mendey, R. Renal traumal *J. Urol. 104:*649, 1970.
12. Thompson, I. M., Latourette, H., Monte, J., et al. Results of nonoperative management of blunt renal trauma. *J. Urol. 118:*522, 1977.
13. Wein, A. J., Murphy, J. J., Mulholland. S. G., et al. A conservative approach to the management of blunt renal trauma. *J. Urol. 117:*425, 1977.
14. Scott, R., Carlton, C. E., and Goldman, M. Penetrating injuries of the kidney: an analysis of 181 patients. *J. Urol. 101:*247, 1969.
15. Griffin, W. O., Jr., Belin, R. P., Ernst, C. B., et al. Intravenous pyelography in abdominal trauma. *J. Trauma 18:*387, 1978.
16. Casgrove, M. D., Mendey, R., and Morrow, J. W. Branch artery ligation for renal arteriovenous fistula. *J. Urol. 110:*632, 1973.
17. Emanuel, B. Weiss, H., and Collin, P. Renal trauma in children. *J. Trauma 17:*275, 1977.
18. Smith, M. J. V., Seidel, R. F., and Bonacarti, A. F. Accident trauma to the kidney in children. *J. Urol. 96:*845, 1966.
19. Persky, L., and Forsythe, W. E. Renal trauma in childhood. *J.A.M.A. 182:*709, 1962.

INDEX